本書是一本用彩圖和文字介紹香港野生和馴化的中草藥書籍
An Illustrated & Descriptive Guide to Medicinal Plants
Indigenous to and Naturalized in Hong Kong with Colored
Plates.

中英對照

香港中草藥 (第七輯)

主 編 者 ....李甯漢　劉啟文

出 版 者 ....商務印書館 (香港) 有限公司
　　　　　　　　　　　香港鰂魚涌芬尼街2號D僑英大廈

印 刷 者 ....中華商務彩色印刷有限公司
　　　　　　　　　　　香港新界大埔汀麗路36號中華商務印刷大廈

版　　次 1997年1月第1版第1次印刷
　　　　　　　　　　　© 1997 商務印書館 (香港) 有限公司
　　　　　　　　　　　ISBN 962 07 3143 3 (精)
　　　　　　　　　　　ISBN 962 07 3144 1 (平)
　　　　　　　　　　　Printed in Hong Kong

香港中草藥

CHINESE MEDICINAL HERBS OF HONG KONG

第七輯 Vol.7

中英對照　CHINESE-ENGLISH

香港中草藥
CHINESE MEDICINAL HERBS OF HONG KONG

第七輯 Vol.7　　李甯漢・劉啟文主編

商務印書館

編輯説明

　　自從我們在1976年7月16日於香港大會堂主辦「香港草藥展覽」迄今，已整整經過二十年。展覽的成功，為《香港中草藥》1至7輯的出版，從人才、組織上準備了條件，也為本港中草藥研究展開了新的一頁。

　　根據《香港植物名錄》（1993年版）記載，香港維管束植物共有2,815種（包括92個變種）。另據我們二十年來的調查研究和1995年5月潘永權先生的統計，香港中草藥共有1,615種，比較我們初時估計的600種多了逾千種。但香港中草藥的一個特點是品種多，然而每一種的蘊藏量卻不多，故此只有大量栽種，才可能提供臨床應用；並必須保護大自然以保留珍貴品種，供繁殖栽培。

　　本輯所載草藥品種中，有8種是我們新發現的香港記錄植物：香港細辛（Asarum hongkongense）、珊瑚薑（Zingiber corallinum）、蘘荷（Zingiber mioga）、陽荷（Zingiber striolatum）、趾葉栝樓（Trichosanthes pedata）、薑黃（Curcuma longa）、藤三七（Anredera cordifolia）和烏藥（Lindera aggregata）等，其中香港細辛是世界上首先在香港發現的植物品種。我們對協助鑑定上述標本的華南植物研究所、香港植物標本室和胡秀英博士等致以衷心的感謝！

　　二十年來，我們堅毅不懈地從事中醫中藥的發揚工作。除編輯《香港中草藥》1至7輯外，並協助香港市政局轄下香港動植物公園和香港漁農處轄下西貢自然教育中心建設兩個中草藥園。從1987年起，參加兩個市政局一年一度於3月舉辦的「香港花卉展覽」，先後十次展出香港中草藥，深受市民歡迎。香港中醫中藥的地位，正日漸受到尊重和承認，同人等深感欣慰。香港豐富的中草藥資源，正待我們發掘整理。古語云：「行百里者，半於九十。」我們今後將再接再厲，繼續努力。

李甯漢　劉啟文
1996年7月16日
於香港中國醫學研究所

《香港中草藥》第7輯編輯委員會

編 輯 顧 問 ： 胡秀英

主　　　　編 ： 李甯漢　劉啟文

副　主　編 ： 吳燕月　劉梅玉

攝　　　影 ： 李甯漢　劉啟文　蔡盤生　林英偉　麥翰雲　何偉琪

翻　　　譯 ： 吳燕月

形態 (中、英文) ： 麥翰雲

編　　　輯 ： 梁澤民　梁安好　李天德　甘長東　蔡盤生　韓碧霞
　　　　　　　潘永權　羅浩林　黎承顯　楊炳成　施濟民　陳展華
　　　　　　　羅惠賢

2

From the Editors

Twenty years have passed since our historic exhibition of Chinese medicinal herbs opening on 16 July, 1976 at the Hong Kong City Hall. Its success ushered in a new page in the study of medicinal herbs in Hong Kong; it also fostered an atmosphere favourable for the gathering of talents, and provided a groundwork for the preparation of the **Chinese Medicinal Herbs of Hong Kong** Volumes 1 to 7.

According to the **Check List of Hong Kong Plants**, 1993 edition, a total of 2,815 plants species (including 92 varietas) exist in Hong Kong. Our study and research over two decades, together with the data compiled by Mr. Poon Wing Kuen, has recorded as many as 1,615 species of Chinese medicinal herbs thriving in Hong Kong —— a thousand species more than our original estimate of 600 species!

Chinese medicinal herbs in Hong Kong are characterized by the fact that an abundant variety exists but in limited quantities. Therefore large scale propagation is necessary to provide for clinical use. In addition, measures should be undertaken to protect the natural environment essential for the conservation of many precious species.

Volume 7 of this book includes 8 newly recorded species of Hong Kong plants discovered by our group. They are: Asarum hongkongense, Zingiber corallinum, Zingiber mioga, Zingiber striolatum, Trichosanthes pedata, Curcuma longa, Anredera cordifolia, and Lindera aggregata, of which the first, Asarum hongkongense, is a new species in the world first discovered in Hong Kong. We are most grateful to experts from the South China Botanical Research Institute, the Hong Kong Herbarium,and Dr. Shiu Ying Hu for their help in identifying the above species.

Over the past twenty years, we have persevered in the study and promotion of Chinese medicinal herbs. Aside from the preparation of the 7 volumes of **Chinese Medicinal Herbs of Hong Kong**, we have also offered assistance and expertise in the establishment of two Chinese medicinal herb gardens —— the first one in the Hong Kong Zoological and Botanical Gardens under the Urban Council, and the second one in the Sai Kung Nature Centre under the Agriculture and Fisheries Department.

Since 1987, we have participated regularly in the annual Hong Kong Flower Show sponsored by the Urban and the Regional Councils in March. Our exhibit of Chinese medicinal herbs has consistently been highly regarded and most popularly received by the local citizens.

We are pleased that traditional Chinese medicine is now receiving increasing respect and recognition in Hong Kong. The rich reserve of Chinese medicinal herbs in Hong Kong is awaiting discovery and study. We shall re-commit ourselves to continue our efforts in this most worthy cause.

Li Ning Hon

Lau Kai Man

Hong Kong Chinese Medical Research Institute

16 July 1996

第七輯目錄

香港中草藥
第七輯

舒　筋　草

Lycopodiastrum casuarinoides (Spring.) Holub.

別　　名　　石子藤、石子藤石松、千金藤、伸筋草、燈籠草。

生長環境　　生於山谷、山坡疏林，常攀於樹上。

採集加工　　藥用全草。全年可採，曬乾或鮮用。

性味功能　　味微甘，性溫。舒筋活血，祛風濕。

主治用法　　1. 風濕關節痛，跌打損傷；2. 月經不調。每用 5 錢至 2 兩，水煎或浸酒服。

方　　例　　治筋骨受傷後屈伸不利：舒筋草1兩，豬筋適量燉服。外用舒筋草2兩，煎水趁熱浸洗患處，並適當運動患肢。

Habitat　　In ravines, woods on slopes, often twining on trees.

Preparation　　Use whole herb. Collect all year round. Dry under sun or use fresh.

Properties　　Mildly sweet tasting; warm. Muscle relaxant; promotes circulation; anti-rheumatic.

Indications　　1. Rheumatic joint pain, traumatic injury; 2. Irregular menses. Use 15-60 gm., as decoction, or steep in wine for oral use.

Prescription　　Post-traumatic contracture: Lycopodium casuarinoides 30 gm., cook with pork tendons for oral consumption. For external use, boil 60 gm. Lycopodium casuarinoides in water for washing the affected parts.

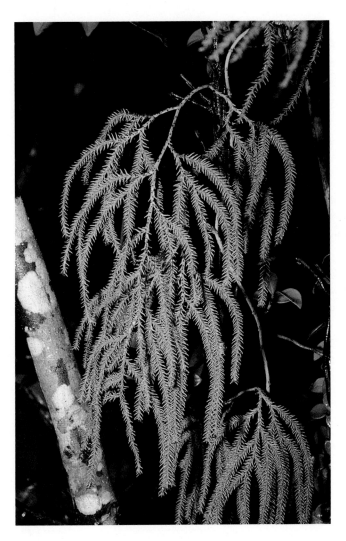

石松科、石松屬之攀援藤本。
莖長達3至4米，基部圓柱狀，直徑
4毫米，上部多2歧分枝。葉小，鑽
狀披針形，稀疏生於主莖上，長5
至 7 毫米，膜質；緊密生於末枝
上，3列，長1.5至3毫米，先端具
1鞭毛。孢子枝較短，2歧分枝，每
枝端具 1 圓柱形略下垂之孢子囊
穗。孢子葉闊卵圓三角形。孢子囊
近圓形。

Lycopodiaceae: A climber, the
primary stem 3-4m long, the basal
portion cylindrical, 4mm across, the
upper portion dichotomously branched.
Leaves small, awl-shaped or lanceolate;
sparsely scattered on the primary stem,
5-7mm long, the upper portion
membranous; those on the ultimate
branches crowded, 3-ranked, two lateral
and one on the other side, awled-shaped,
1.5-3mm long, flagellate at the apex.
Sporagiophore branches shorter,
dichotomously branched, each ultimate
branch terminated by a cylindrical
strobile; sporophylls broad-ovate or
orbiculate-deltoid. Sporangia spherical.

單葉新月蕨

Pronephrium simplex (Hk.) Holttum

別　　名　草鞋青、新月蕨、蛇皮草、鵝仔草。

生長環境　生於林下或溪邊陰濕地。

採集加工　藥用全草。全年可採，曬乾或鮮用。

性味功能　味甘、微澀，性涼。清熱解毒，消滯。

主　　治　1. 扁桃體炎；2. 消化不良，痢疾；3. 蛇咬傷。每用5錢，水煎服。外用適量鮮品搗敷患處。

方　　例　1. 扁桃體炎：單葉新月蕨1兩，水煎，沖酒含服。

2. 蛇咬傷：單葉新月蕨5錢，續隨子草5分，水煎服。外用鮮品適量搗敷患處。

Habitat　　Under woods or damp soil along streams.

Preparation　　Use whole herb. Collect all year round, dry under sun or use fresh.

Properties　　Sweet and mildly astringent tasting; cold. Anti-inflammatory; promotes digestion.

Indications　　1. Tonsillitis; 2. Indigestion, dysentery; 3. Snake bites. Use 15 gm., as decoction. Mash fresh herb for external use.

Prescriptions　　1. Tonsillitis: Pronephrium simplex 30 gm., as decoction. Take with wine and swallow slowly.

2. Snake bites: Pronephrium simplex 15 gm., Euphorbia lathyris 1.5 gm., as decoction. Mash fresh herb as poultice.

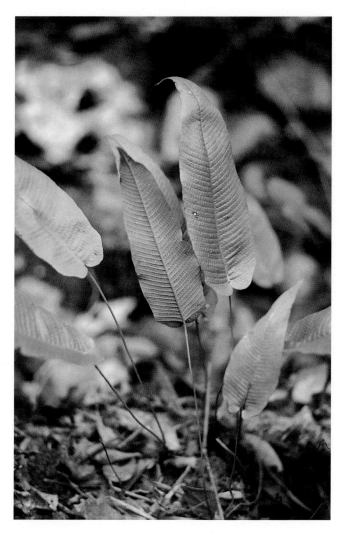

　　金星蕨科、新月蕨屬。植株高可達 40 厘米。根狀莖細長，橫走，頂端有疏鱗片。葉遠生，二型，單一；不育葉紙質，乾後仍為綠色，橢圓狀披針形，葉基心形或偶有一對耳片，全緣或具粗鈍齒，葉脈網狀，在側脈間形成兩行整齊的方形網眼，葉柄幼長，禾稈色。可育葉高出不育葉，葉柄更長，葉片披針形，葉基心形或戟形。孢子囊羣生於小脈上，延漸伸展而生滿於葉底面；孢子囊羣幼時圓形，無蓋。

Thelypteridaceae: Ferns up to 40cm high. Rhizomes slender, long-creeping, with sparse terminal scales. Fronds simple, dimorphous. Sterile leaves papery, remaining green when dry, elliptical-lanceolate, base cordate or occasionally with one pair of auricles, margins entire or roughly dentate, veins reticulate, forming two columns of tidy square areoles between the lateral veins, stipes slender and long, straw-coloured. Fertile leaves longer than the sterile ones, stipes also longer; laminae lanceolate, base cordate or hastate. Sori round when young, exindusiate, occurring on veinlets, extending gradually over the undersurface.

瓦　韋

Lepisorus thunbergianus (Kaulf.) Ching

別　　名　劍丹、骨牌草、落星草、金雞尾。

生長環境　生於巖石或樹幹上。

採集加工　藥用全草。夏、秋採收，曬乾。

性味功能　味苦，性寒。清熱，利尿。

主治用法　1. 尿路感染，尿血；2. 口腔炎，扁桃體炎；3. 結膜炎，角膜炎；4. 支氣管炎，咳血。每用5錢至1兩，水煎服。外用治瘡癤，鮮品搗敷患處。

方　　例　1. 尿路感染：瓦韋、車前草各1兩，水煎服。

2. 口腔炎，扁桃體炎：瓦韋、忍冬藤各1兩，水煎服。

3. 結膜炎，角膜炎：瓦韋1兩，谷精草5錢，水煎服。

主要成分　含蛻皮甾酮（ecdysterone），為一種昆蟲變態激素。

附　　註　本品對金黃色葡萄球菌、傷寒桿菌、綠膿桿菌、弗氏痢疾桿菌有抑制作用。

Habitat　　　On rocks and tree trunks.

Preparation　　Use whole herb. Collect in summer and autumn, dry under sun.

Properties　　Bitter tasting; cold. Anti-inflammatory, diuretic.

Indications　　1. Urinary tract infection, hematuria; 2. Stomatitis, tonsillitis; 3. Conjunctivitis, keratitis; 4. Bronchitis; haemoptysis. Use 15-30 gm., as decoction. External use in furuncles by applying mashed fresh herb to lesion.

Prescriptions　　1. Urinary tract infection: Lepisorus thunbergianus, Plantago major, 30 gm. each, as decoction.

2. Stomatitis, tonsillitis: Lepisorus thunbergianus, Lonicera japonica vines, 30 gm. each, as decoction.

3. Conjunctivitis, keratitis: Lepisorus thunbergianus 30 gm., Eriocaulon sexangulare 15 gm., as decoction.

Remarks　　The herb contains ecdysterone, a mutant hormone of insects. This herb is bacteriostatic against Staph. aureus, typhoid bacilli, Pseudomonas, and Shigella.

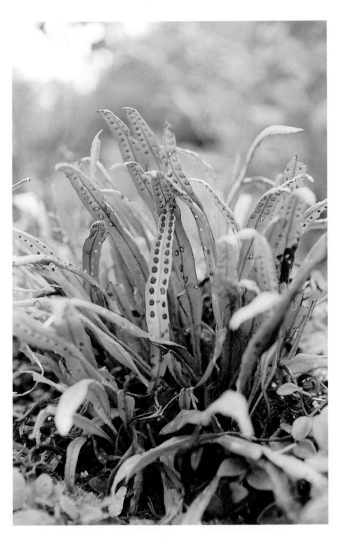

　　水龍骨科、瓦韋屬之蕨類植物，植株高約20厘米。橫走之根狀莖密生鱗片，鱗片黑色，邊緣有齒。葉片長條狀披針形，革質，每片垂直生於根莖上；有短葉柄或幾無柄；除主脈外，葉脈不明顯。孢子囊羣直徑約3毫米，沿着主脈呈兩列排列，囊羣間頗靠近。

Polypodiaceae: Ferns; perennial herbs, 20cm high. Rhizome creeping, densely covered with dentate black scales. Fronds linear lanceolate, coriaceous, arising vertically from the rhizome, stipes short or sessile, veins inconspicuous except the mid-rib. Sori 3mm in diameter, arranged into two rows along either side of the mid-rib, quite close together.

青　蔞

Piper betle L.

別　　名　　蔞葉、青蒟、檳榔蔞、土蓽撥、蒟醬、浮留藤、蔞藤。

生長環境　　多為栽培。

採集加工　　藥用全株及果實。莖葉全年可採，果實秋後成熟時採，曬乾。

性味功能　　味辛、微甘，性溫。祛風，健胃，化痰，消腫，止癢。

主治用法　　1. 風寒咳嗽，支氣管哮喘；2. 胃寒痛；3. 風濕骨痛。每用1至3錢，水煎服。外用治皮膚濕疹、腳癬，適量煎水外洗或浸泡患處。

方　　例　　風寒咳嗽：蔞葉 7 片，北杏仁 3 錢，瘦豬肉 4 兩，水煎服。

主要成分　　葉含揮發油，成分有胡椒酚（chavicol）、蔞葉酚（chavibetol）等。

Habitat　　Mostly cultivated.

Preparation　　Use whole herb and fruits. Leaves and stems can be harvested all year round. Fruits are collected in autumn when ripe and dried under sun.

Properties　　Acrid and slightly sweet tasting; neutral. Dispels chill, reduced swelling; stomachic, expectorant, anti-pruritic.

Indications　　1. Colds and coughs, asthmatic bronchitis; 2. Stomach discomfort; 3. Rheumatic bone pain. Use 3-10 gm., as decoction. Also useful externally in eczema, ringworm infection of feet, by boiling the herb in water for washing or soaking the affected part.

Prescription　　Colds and coughs: Use 7 Piper betle leaves, Prunus armeniaca seeds 10 gm., boil with 120 gm. of lean pork in water and consume.

Remarks　　Contains volatile oil, chavicol and chavibetol.

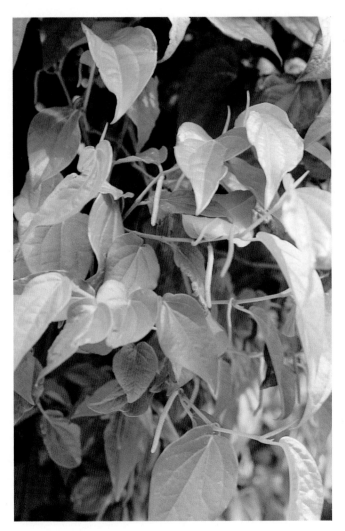

胡椒科、胡椒屬之藤本，近木質，長數米，節上常生根。葉互生，革質，寬卵形或心形，有時葉片左右不對稱，長6至15厘米，葉基心形或斜歪的淺心形；葉柄長2至5厘米。雌雄異株，穗狀花序，無花被；雄花序長約9厘米，下垂；總花梗較短；苞片圓形，盾狀，有短柄，柄上有毛；雄蕊2；雌花序長1.5至3.5厘米，子房嵌生於肉質的花序軸的凹陷處，並與之合生；柱頭4至5。漿果與花序軸合生成肉質果穗。花期：五月至七月。

Piperaceae: Sublignified vines, several m long, nodes often producing roots. Leaves alternate, leathery, ovate or cordate, occasionally oblique, 6-15cm long, base cordate or obliquely subcordate, petioles 2-5cm long. Flowers unisexual, dioecious, in slender spikes, apetalous; male spikes 9cm long, pendulous, peduncle short, bracts orbicular, peltate, on short hairy stalk, stamens 2; female spikes 1.5-3.5cm long, ovary sunken into the fleshy axis and adnate to it, stigmas 4 or 5. Berries adnate to the fleshy axis. Flowering from May to July.

梨 果 榕

Ficus pyriformis Hook. et Arn.

別　　名　舶梨榕、水石榴、梨狀牛奶子。

生長環境　生於山澗邊灌木叢中。

採集加工　藥用莖。全年可採，曬乾或鮮用。

性味功能　味澀，性涼。清熱，利尿，止痛。

主治用法　1. 腎炎，膀胱炎，尿道炎；2. 腎性水腫，心性水腫；3. 胃痛。每用 5 錢至 1 兩，水煎服。

Habitat　　　In thickets along sides of creeks.

Preparation　Use stem. Collect all year round, dry under sun or use fresh.

Properties　Astringent tasting; cool. Anti-inflammatory, diuretic, analgesic.

Indications　1. Nephritis, cystitis, urethritis; 2. Nephrotic edema, cardiac edema; 3. Epigastric pain. Use 15-30 gm., as decoction.

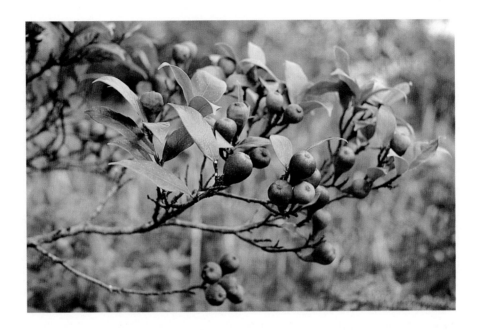

　　桑科、無花果屬之灌木，高1至2米；枝多分枝，植株常呈半平臥狀。葉互生；葉型3款：倒卵形、披針形及卵圓形；葉尖為延長之急尖；主脈凸起；葉柄短。無花果梨形；單生於葉腋；嫩時綠色，熟時紅或深紫色；成熟之花序托成厚乾之海綿狀壁；雌果較瘦果大。雄花及瘦花同生於瘦果內；雌花生於雌果內，雌花果壁脹大成氣囊狀軟墊，內藏種子。種子近球形。花期：四月至六月。

Moracea: Shrub 1-2m high, branches many divided, sometimes semi-prostrate. Leaves alternate, leaf shape three forms: obovate, lanceolate and elliptical, all with an elongate acuminate tip, midrib raised, petiole short. Figs pyriform in shape, borne singly in leaf axils, green when young, red or dark purple when mature; ripe syconium becomes a thick dry spongy wall; female fig larger than gall fig. Male flowers and gall flowers borne together in gall fig, female flowers in female fig. Female flower pericarp swollen to form an alveolar cushion around the near-spherical seeds. Flowering from April to June.

青 皮 樹

Schoepfia chinensis Gardn. et Champ.

別　　名　華南青皮木、青皮木、華青皮木、管花青皮木、碎骨木。

生長環境　生於山谷密林中。

採集加工　藥用根、樹枝及葉。根及樹枝全年可採，夏、秋採葉，切碎曬乾或鮮用。

性味功能　味甘、淡，性涼。清熱利濕，消腫止痛。

主治用法　根：治急性黃疸型肝炎。每用5錢至1兩，水煎服。樹枝及葉：1. 風濕痺痛；2. 跌打損傷，骨折。每用1至2兩，水煎服或煎水外洗；另用鮮枝葉搗爛敷患處。

Habitat　　In valleys and thick woods.

Preparation　　Use roots, stems, and leaves. Collect roots and stems all year round, collect leaves in autumn, cut fine and dry under sun, or use fresh.

Properties　　Sweet, bland tasting; cool. Anti-inflammatory, diuretic; reduces swelling; analgesic.

Indications　　Roots: Acute icteric hepatitis, use 15-30 gm., as decoction. Stems and leaves: 1. Rheumatism; 2. Traumatic injury, fractures. Use 30-60 gm., as decoction, or boil in water for washing. Mash fresh herb for topical application.

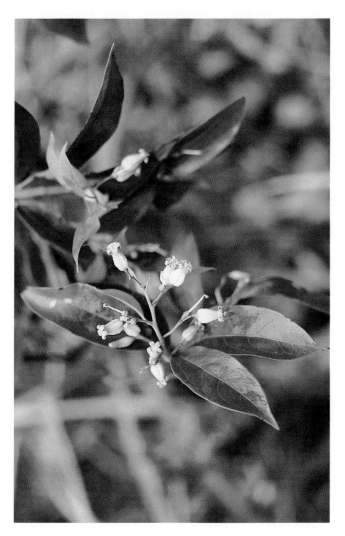

鐵青樹科、青皮木屬之落葉灌木，高約 2 至 5 米。葉互生，堅紙質，狹橢圓形至矩圓狀披針形。聚傘花序腋生，長約 2 厘米，通常具 3 朵花；花芳香，無柄；花萼杯狀，大部分與子房合生，宿存；花冠筒狀，筒頂 4 至 5 裂，裂片細小，內面近花藥處生 1 束絲狀體；雄蕊與花冠裂片同數，無退化雄蕊；子房半下位，柱頭 3 裂，不伸出於花冠筒之外。核果橢圓形，成熟時紅色或紫紅色。花期：二月至四月。

Olacaceae: Deciduous shrubs 2-5m high. Leaves alternate, firm papery, narrow elliptic to oblong-lanceolate. Flowers fragrant, sessile, usually 3-flowered in axillary cymes which are 2cm long; calyx cupular, mostly connate with ovary, persistent; corolla tubular, limb 4-5 lobed, lobes small, bearing on the inside a tuft of hairs near the anthers; stamens equal limb lobes in number, without staminodes; semi-inferior ovary, stigma 3-lobed, not exceeding beyond the corolla tube. Drupes elliptic, red or scarlet at maturity. Flowering from February to April.

五 瓣 寄 生

Helixanthera parasitica Lour.

別　　名　離瓣寄生、五瓣桑寄生、桂花寄生、木棉寄生。

生長環境　常寄生於油茶、山茶科、樟科、大戟科等植物上。

採集加工　藥用全株。全年可採，曬乾。

性味功能　化痰，止咳，祛風濕。

主治用法　1. 肺結核，咳嗽；2. 風濕痹痛；3. 痢疾。每用 3 至 5 錢，水煎服。

附　　註　寄生類植物與寄主有密切關係，如寄生在有毒植物上，不宜使用！

Habitat　　Often parasitic on plants belonging to the tea, cinnamon, or euphorbia families (Theaceae, Lauraceae, Euphorbiaceae).

Preparation　　Use whole herb. Collect all year round, dry under sun.

Properties　　Expectorant, antitussive, anti-rheumatic.

Indications　　1. Pulmonary tuberculosis, coughs; 2. Rheumatic pains; 3. Dysentery. Use 10-15 gm., as decoction.

Remarks　　Parasitic plants have close relationship with their hosts; therefore do not use those plants which are parasitic on poisonous hosts.

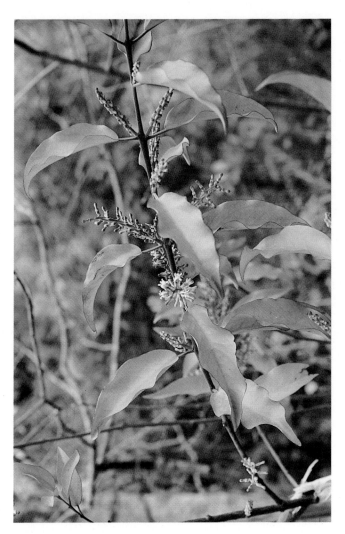

　　桑寄生科、離瓣寄生屬之灌
木，高約 1.5 米。嫩莖表面皮滑，
質略軟，呈披散狀。葉對生，紙質
或薄革質；卵形至卵狀披針形；葉
頂端急尖至漸尖，葉基闊楔形至近
圓形；兩面之側脈明顯。總狀花
序，1 至 2 個腋生或生於小枝已落葉
之腋部；花紅色、淡紅色或淡黃
色，被暗褐色或灰色乳頭狀毛；花
蕾時花冠之下半部膨脹，具 5 條拱
起的棱；花瓣 5 片，上半部反折。
果紅色，被乳頭狀毛。花期：二月
至四月。

Loranthaceae: Shrubs
approximately 1.5m high. Young stems
glabrous, soft, spreading. Leaves
opposite, papery or thin-leathery, ovate
to ovate-lanceolate, apex acute or
acuminate, base broad cuneate or
suborbicular, lateral veins on both
surfaces prominent. Racemes 1 to 2
borne in leaf axils. Flowers red, pink or
light-yellow, covered with dark brown
or grey papillae. When in bud the corolla
swells at the lower part of the flower bud,
with 5 elevated ridges; petals 5, upper
part recurved. Fruit red, with papillae.
Flowering from February to April.

香 港 細 辛

Asarum hongkongense S. M. Hwang et T. P. Wong

生長環境　生於山坡灌木林陰下多石、潮濕而排水良好之泥土中。

採集加工　藥用根或全草。全年可採，陰乾或鮮用。

性味功能　味苦、辛，性溫。有小毒。散寒，止咳，止痛。

主治用法　1. 風寒咳嗽，痰多稀白；2. 風濕關節痛。每用5分至1錢，水煎服。外用治牙痛，跌打腫痛，適量煎水含漱，或鮮品搗敷患處。

附　　註　香港細辛是世界上首先在香港發現的新品種。本品辛味較弱，功效亦遜於正細辛（Asarum sieboldii Mig.）。

Habitat　In moist and stony soil with good drainage under shaded thickets on hilly slopes.

Preparation　Use roots or whole herb. Collect all year round, dry under shade or use fresh.

Properties　Acrid tasting; warm. Slightly poisonous. Dispels "coldness" ntitussive, analgesic.

Indications　1. Coughs, excessive sputum; 2. Rheumatic arthralgia. Use 1.5-3 gm., as decoction. External use in toothache, traumatic injury. Boil suitable amount of the herb in water for gargle, or use fresh herb as poultice.

Remarks　Asarum hongkongense was first in the world to be discovered in Hong Kong. This herb has a weaker acrid taste and is also weaker in efficacy than the traditionally used A. sieboldii Mig.

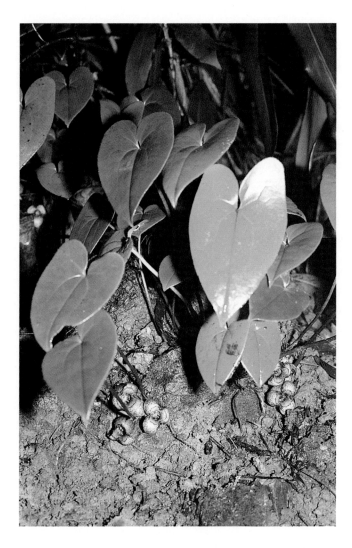

馬兜鈴科之多年生爬行草本。根狀莖長，3毫米粗；根2毫米直徑，近肉質；根及莖均有明顯辛辣氣及味。葉近革質，卵狀心形；葉尖急尖或短尖頭，葉基心形；葉緣稍背捲，具緣毛或細鋸齒；葉面光亮；基出脈5至7，在葉背隆起；葉柄長。花單生，罈形；淡黃綠色，上有無數深紫點，成熟尤深色；花被筒寬卵形，內有縱向皺紋；檐3裂，裂片寬卵形，反捲；雄蕊12；花柱6。花期：冬、春二季。

Aristolochiaceae: Perennial creeping herbs. Rhizomes long, 3 mm in diameter; roots 2 mm in diameter, subcarnose; both with strongly pungent odour and taste. Leaves subcoriaceous; ovate-cordate; apex acute or mucronate, base cordate; margin slightly rolling downwards, tomentose or crenulate; glossy above; primary nerves 5, occasionally 7, elevated beneath; petioles long. Flowers solitary, campanulate; tinged yellow with numerous dark purple puncta, darker at maturity; perianth tube broadly ovoid, with longitudinal verrucose wrinkles inside, limb 3-lobed, broadly ovate, recurved; stamens 12; styles 6. Flowering in winter and spring.

藤 三 七

Anredera cordifolia (Tenore) Steenis

別　　名　土三七、心葉落葵薯、落葵薯、藤子三七。

生長環境　多為栽培，或逸生於村邊林下。

採集加工　藥用藤及珠芽，塊根可食。全年可採，曬乾或鮮用。

性味功能　味微苦，性溫。滋補強壯，消腫散瘀。

主治用法　1. 病後體弱；2. 腰膝痺痛。每用 1 至 2 兩，水煎服。外用治跌打損傷、骨折，風濕性關節炎。鮮品適量，搗爛敷患處。

方　　例　病後體弱，腰膝痺痛：藤三七 2 兩，適量雞或豬肉燉服，服湯食肉。

附　　註　藤三七原產美洲熱帶地區。是香港新記錄植物。

Habitat　　Mostly cultivated, or occasionally found on village edges or under woods as escapes.

Preparation　　Use roots and small shoots. Tubers are edible. Collect all year round, dry under sun or use fresh.

Properties　　Slightly bitter tasting, warm. Tonic, reduces swelling and haematoma.

Indications　　1. Debility after illness; 2. Loin and knee pains and numbness. Use 30-60 gm., as decoction. External use in traumatic injury, fractures, rheumatic arthritis, mash herb as poultice.

Prescription　　Debility after illness, knee and loin pains: Anredera cordifolia 60 gm., cook with suitable amount of pork or chicken as soup dish.

Remarks　　Anredera cordifolia originated in the American tropics. It is a newly recorded species in Hong Kong.

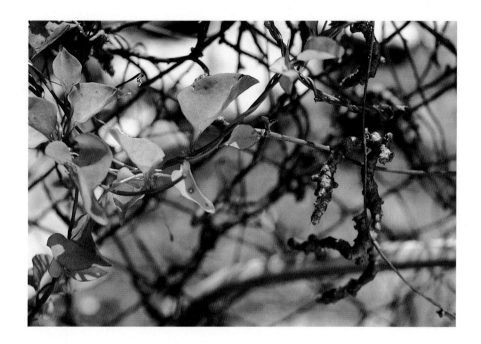

　　落葵科、落葵薯屬之多年生草質藤本，具塊根。莖醬紅色，右旋纏繞，長可達3米，具球狀珠芽。葉卵狀心臟形，互生，葉柄長度較葉片略長。總狀花序長可達25厘米，總花軸淡紅色；花白色，細小，芳香；花萼2片，圓形；花冠5片，卵狀長圓形且略內捲；雄蕊5，花絲在花蕾內反折；花萼、花冠、花絲三者合生成杯狀；子房上位。果球形，包藏於宿存的花冠筒內。花期：八月。

Basellaceae: Perennial herbal vines, with root-tubers. Stems reddish-caramel, twining right-handed, up to 3m long, bearing globular bulbils. Leaves alternate, ovate-cordate, petioles longer than the laminae. Inflorescence in the form of racemes which may reach a length of 25cm, rachis pinkish, flowers white, small, fragrant, sepals 2, orbicular; corolla 5-lobed, ovate, slightly rolling inwards; stamens 5, filaments reflexed; calyx, corolla and filaments connate, cupular; ovary superior. Fruits globular, borne inside the persistent corolla tube. Flowering in August.

毛柱鐵綫蓮 (甘草藤)

Clematis meyeniana Walp.

別　　名　南鐵綫蓮、吹風藤、老虎鬚藤、威靈仙。

生長環境　生於山坡、路旁灌木叢中。

採集加工　藥用根、莖。全年可採，曬乾。

性味功能　味辛、鹹，性溫。有小毒。祛風濕，活血止痛。

主治用法　1. 風濕痹痛，肢體麻木，屈伸不利；2. 骨哽咽喉；3. 跌打瘀痛。每用 2 至 3 錢，水煎服。

附　　註　本品功效與威靈仙 (Clematis chinensis) 相似。

Habitat　　On slopes and among roadside bushes.

Preparation　　Use roots and stems. Collect all year round, dry under sun.

Properties　　Acrid and salty tasting; warm. Slightly poisonous. Anti-rheumatic; promotes circulation; analgesic.

Indications　　1. Rheumatic pains, numbness, impaired mobility; 2. Bone stuck in throat; 3. Traumatic bruises. Use 5-10 gm., as decoction.

Remarks　　The therapeutic effects are similar to those of Clematis chinensis.

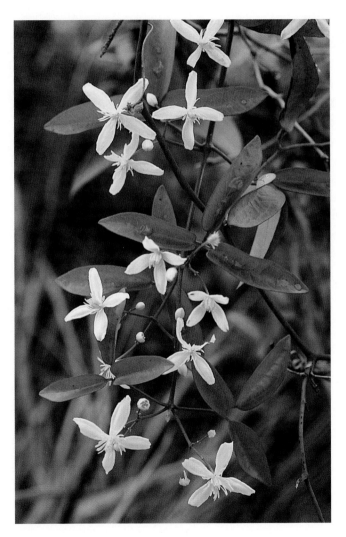

毛茛科、鐵綫蓮屬之多年生木質藤本。老莖圓柱形，有縱條紋，幼莖有棱。葉對生，近革質；3出複葉，小葉片卵形或卵狀圓形，有時為寬卵形，葉尖銳尖或漸尖，葉基圓形或寬楔形，全緣；葉柄及小葉柄常伸長而纏繞於其他物體之上。圓錐狀聚傘花序，腋生或頂生，花多數，花序長；苞片小；萼片4，白色，長橢圓形或披針形，花瓣狀，外面有絨毛。果鐮刀狀狹卵形或狹倒卵形，有柔毛，具宿存之花柱。花期：七月。

Ranunculaceae: Annual woody vines. Old stems cylindrical, with longitudinal striations; young stems with ridges. Leaves opposite, subcoriaceous; trifoliolate, leaflets ovate, ovate-orbicular or broad ovate; apex acute or acuminate, cuneate at base; entire, petiole or petiolule often extended to twine on other objects. Flowers numerous, in axillary or terminal paniculate cymes, inflorescence long; bracts small; sepals 4, whitish, oblong-elliptic or lanceolate, petaloid, tomentose on the outside. Fruits narrow falcate-ovate or narrow obovate, pilose, with persistent styles. Flowering in July.

蒼白秤鈎風

Diploclisia glaucescens (Bl.) Diels

別　　名　秤鈎風、穿牆風、土防己。

生長環境　生於疏林或灌木叢中。

採集加工　藥用藤、葉。全年可採，鮮用或曬乾備用。

性味功能　味微苦，性寒。清熱利濕，消腫解毒。

主治用法　1. 風濕骨痛；2. 膽囊炎；3. 尿路感染；4. 毒蛇咬傷。每用3至5錢，水煎服。治毒蛇咬傷同時用鮮葉搗爛，外敷傷口周圍。

主要成分　根、藤含生物鹼。

Habitat　　Among sparse woods or shrubs.

Preparation　Use vines and leaves. Collect all year round, use fresh or dry under sun.

Properties　Slighty bitter tasting; cold. Anti-inflammatory, diuretic; relieves swelling.

Indications　1. Rheumatic bone pain; 2. Cholecysitiis; 3. Urinary tract infection; 4. Snake bites. Use 10-15 gm., as decoction. In snake bites, may also mash fresh herb and apply externally as poultice around wound.

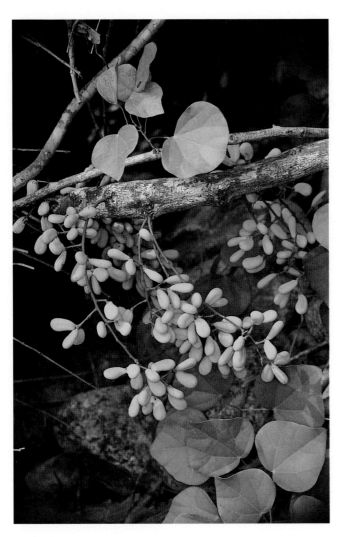

　　防己科、秤鈎風屬之多年生木質藤本。莖上具細條紋。葉紙質至革質，寬卵形，5 出基脈，葉緣輕微波浪形，葉底面粉綠色，底面大葉脈凸起；葉柄約與葉片等長。雌雄異株；聚傘狀圓錐花序生於老莖上；雌及雄花序長可達 20 厘米；雄花 6 數，花萼片淡黃色而夾有黑色斑紋，花瓣寬倒卵形；雌花具心皮 3，退化雄蕊 6。核果倒卵狀矩圓形，具白色粉末。花期：春季。

Menispermaceae: Perennial woody vines. Stems with small stripes. Leaves papery to leathery, broad ovate, pentanervious, margins slightly undulate, lower surface whitish-green, mid-ribs elevated on lower surfaces; petioles almost equal laminae in length. Dioecious; cymous-paniculate inflorescence emerges from old stems, with both male and female ones reaching a length of up to 20cm; male flowers 6-merous, sepals pale-yellow with black mottles, petals broad-obovate; female flowers with three carpels and six staminodes. Fruits obovate-oblong, drupe, covered by a white powdery bloom. Flowering in spring.

糞 箕 篤

Stephania longa Lour.

別　　名　千金藤、三角藤、犁壁藤。

生長環境　生於山地、疏林中，常纏繞於灌木上。

採集加工　藥用全株。全年可採，曬乾或鮮用。

性味功能　味微苦、澀，性平。清熱解毒，利尿消腫。

主治用法　1. 腎盂腎炎，膀胱炎，慢性腎炎；2. 腸炎，痢疾；3. 風濕疼痛，腰腿痛；4. 毒蛇咬傷，瘡癤，化膿性中耳炎。每用5錢至1兩，水煎服。孕婦忌服。外用適量，鮮品搗敷患處，或用藥液滴耳。

主要成分　根和莖含生物鹼，總鹼含量達 0.86 %。其中含千金藤醇靈（stephanoline）、糞箕篤鹼（longanine）、輪環藤寧鹼、高阿莫靈鹼等。

Habitat　　　　On hilly areas and in woods, often twining on shrubs.

Preparation　　Use whole herb. Collect all year round, dry under sun or use fresh.

Properties　　Slightly bitter and astringent tasting; neutral. Anti-inflammatory, diuretic; reduces swelling.

Indications　　1. Pyelonephritis, cystitis, chronic nephritis; 2. Enteritis, dysentery; 3. Rheumatism, lumbago; 4. Poisonous snake bites, furunculosis, purulent otitis media. Use 15-30 gm., as decoction. Contraindicated in pregnancy. For external use, mash suitable amount of fresh herb for topical application, or use juice extract as ear drops.

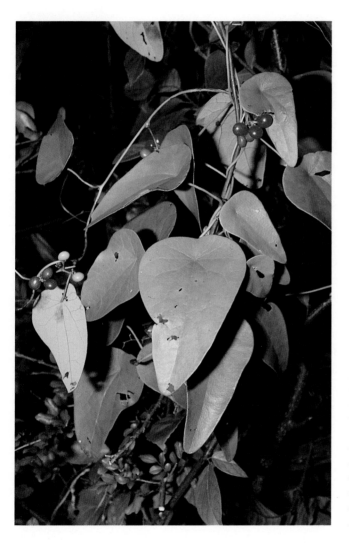

防己科、千金藤屬纏繞藤本，長1至4米。葉紙質，互生，三角狀卵形，長3至9厘米，寬2至6厘米，全緣而背捲，頂端鈍，或具小凸尖，葉基截形或微凹，掌狀脈9至11條；葉柄長，盾狀着生。花單性，雌雄異株；雄花序柔弱，傘形至聚傘形，萼片6至8，花瓣4，有時3，聚藥雄蕊長約0.6毫米；雌花序較粗壯，萼片4，花瓣4。核果成熟時紅色。花期：四月至八月。

Menispermaceae: Twining vines, 1-4m long. Leaves papery, alternate, ovate-deltoid, 3-9cm long by 2-6cm wide, attached to a long petiole in a peltate manner, margin entire and reflexed underneath; apex obtuse or mucronate, base truncate or slightly concave, palmate veins 9 to 11. Flowers unisexual, dioecious; male inflorescence slender, simple to compound umbelliform, calyx 6-8 lobed, petals 4, occasionally 3, synandrium approx. 0.6mm long; female inflorescence more stout, calyx lobes and petals both 4; drupes red when mature. Flowering from April to August.

天　竺　桂

Cinnamomum japonicum Sieb.

別　　名　土肉桂、土桂皮、山肉桂、月桂、竺香。

生長環境　生於山坡樹林中。

採集加工　藥用樹皮、根、枝葉。冬季採樹皮，陰乾。

性味功能　味辛，性溫。袪寒鎮痛，行氣健胃。

主治用法　1. 胃腹寒痛；2. 風濕痛；3. 創傷出血。每用 1 至 2 錢，水煎服。陰虛火盛者忌用。

主要成分　樹皮含揮發油約 1%，油中含水芹烯、丁香酚、甲基丁香酚（methyl eugenol）。葉含揮發油約 1%，油中含黃樟醚約 60%、丁香酚約 3% 及 1,8- 按葉素等。

附　　註　本品功用似肉桂（C. cassia），但其皮薄力弱，功效遠遜肉桂，一般供香料或調味料用，或用葉、樹皮提煉芳香油作殺菌藥劑。

Habitat　　　In woods on slopes.

Preparation　Use bark, roots, branches and leaves. Collect bark in winter, dry in shade.

Properties　Acrid tasting; warm. Analgesic; promotes "qi" circulation; stomachic.

Indications　1. Gastric and abdominal pain; 2. Rheumatic pain; 3. Wound bleeding. Use 3-5 gm., as decoction. Contraindicated in cases of "Yin" deficiency accompanied by "Fire" excesses (with symptoms like flushed cheeks and irritability).

Remarks　This herb has similar action as C. cassia, but the bark is thinner, and action is far weaker. It is usually used as a spice.

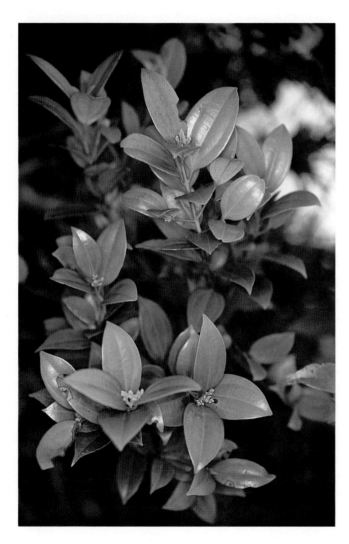

樟科、樟屬之常綠高大喬木，高可達 15 米。枝條細弱，紅或紅褐色，具香氣。葉長圓狀披針形，革質；葉面光亮綠色，葉背晦暗灰綠色；離基 3 出脈，3 脈均向表背面隆起；葉柄紅褐色。圓錐花序腋生，末端為 3 至 5 朵花的聚傘花序，花細小；花被筒倒錐狀，花被裂片 6，卵圓形，先端尖。能育雄蕊 9，花絲被柔毛，第 3 輪花絲有一對腎形腺體；柱頭盤狀。果長圓形，果托淺杯狀。花期：四月。

Lauraceae: Large evergreen trees, up to 15m high. Branches weak; red or reddish-brown; aromatic. Leaves oblong-lanceolate, leathery; glossy green above, dull grey-green beneath; trinervious, elevated on the underside; petioles reddish-brown. Flowers minute, 3-5 flowered cymes forming into axillary panicles; perianth-tube obconic, 6-lobed, ovate, apex pointed. Fertile stamens 9, filaments pilose, the third whorl of filaments with a pair of reniform glands; stigma disc-shaped.Fruits oblong, receptacle shallowly cupular. Flowering in April.

烏　藥

Lindera aggregata (Sims) Kosterm.

別　　名　　天台烏藥、台烏、香葉子樹、旁其、矮樟。

生長環境　　生於向陽山坡灌木林中。

採集加工　　藥用根、樹皮。冬春採挖，切片，曬乾。

性味功能　　味辛，性溫。溫中健胃，理氣止痛。

主治用法　　1.胃氣痛，吐瀉腹痛；2.痛經，疝痛；3.膀胱虛冷，遺尿，尿頻；4.風濕疼痛，跌打傷痛。每用 1 至 3 錢，水煎服。外用治外傷出血，研末外敷。

方　　例　　1.胃痛，吐瀉腹痛：烏藥、青木香各 3 錢，水煎服。

2. 膀胱虛冷，遺尿，尿頻：烏藥、益智仁、淮山各 3 錢，水煎服。

3. 痛經：烏藥、香附、生薑各 3 錢，砂仁、木香各 2 錢，水煎服。

主要成分　　根含揮發油 0.1-0.2%，成分為龍腦、檸檬烯、α 及 β 葎草烯等。

附　　註　　烏藥是香港新記錄植物。

Habitat　　In thickets on sunny slopes.

Preparation　　Use roots and bark. Collect in winter and spring, slice, dry under sun.

Properties　　Acrid tasting; warm. Stomachic, analgesic.

Indications　　1. Stomach discomfort, vomiting; 2. Dysmenorrhea, hernial pain; 3. Urinary incontinence, frequency; 4. Rheumatic pain, traumatic injury. Use 3-10 gm., as decoction. External use in wound bleeding, mash herb for local application.

Prescriptions　　1. Gastric pain and discomfort, diarrhea and vomiting: Lindera aggregata, Aristolochia debilis roots, 10 gm. each, as decoction.

2. Presence of "cold" in the urinary bladder, exhibiting itself as enuresis and frequent urination: Lindera aggregata, Alpinia oxyphylla fruits, Dioscorea opposita, 10 gm. each, as decoction.

3. Dysmenorrhea: Lindera aggregata, Cyperus rotundus rhizomes, Zingiber officinale, 10 gm. each, Amomum villosum fruits, Aucklandia lappa roots, 6 gm. each, as decoction.

Remarks　　Lindera aggregata is a newly recorded spiecies in Hong Kong.

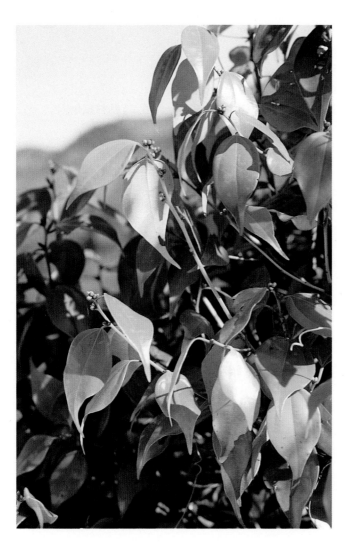

　　樟科、釣樟屬之常綠灌木或小
喬木，高約 5 米。樹皮灰綠色，嫩
莖密生鏽色毛。葉互生，革質，橢
圓形、卵形或近圓形；葉頂端長漸
尖或短尾尖；葉面有光澤，葉背密
生灰白色柔毛；3出脈；葉柄短。雌
雄異株；傘形花序腋生，總花梗極
短或無；花被片6，淡綠色；能育
雄蕊9，花藥2室，均內向瓣裂。果
實橢圓形，熟時黑色。花期：三月
至四月。

Lauraceae: Evergreen shrubs or
small trees, about 5m high. Bark grey-
green, young stems densely rust-
coloured pilose. Leaves alternate,
leathery, elliptic, ovate or suborbicular;
apex acuminate or mucronate; glossy
above, with dense grey-white
pubescence underneath; triplinervious;
petioles short. Dioecious; umbels
axillary, peduncles very short or absent;
perianth 6-lobed, light-green; fertile
stamens 9, anthers 2-celled, both splitting
valvate inwards. Fruits elliptic, black at
maturity. Flowering from March to
April.

豺 皮 樟

Litsea rotundifolia Hemsl. var. oblongifolia (Nees) Allen

別　　名　白葉仔、白柴、大灰木、圓葉木薑子、豺皮黃肉楠。

生長環境　生於山坡灌木林中。

採集加工　藥用根。全年可採，切片，陰乾或鮮用。

性味功能　味辛，性溫。祛風濕，活血，止痛。

主治用法　1.風濕關節痛，腰腿痛；2.胃痛，經痛；3.腹瀉，水腫；4.跌打損傷。每用 5 錢至 1 兩，水煎或浸酒服。

主要成分　葉顯黃酮甙、酚類、氨基酸反應。莖皮顯生物鹼反應。根含生物鹼、酚類、氨基酸。

Habitat　　In thickets on slopes.

Preparation　　Use roots. Collect all year round, slice, dry in shade or use fresh.

Properties　　Acrid tasting; warm. Anti-rheumatic; promotes circulation; analgesic.

Indications　　Rheumatic arthralgia, lumbago; 2. Epigastric pain, dysmenorrhea; 3. Diarrhea, edema; 4. Traumatic injury. Use 15-30 gm., as decoction, or steep in wine for oral use.

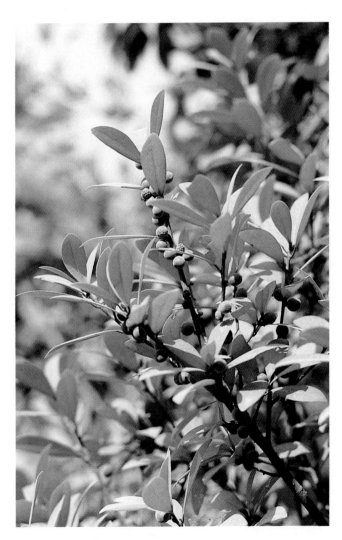

　　樟科、木薑子屬之常綠灌木或
小喬木。葉互生，革質；葉片卵狀
長圓形，先端鈍或短漸尖，基部楔
形或鈍；葉面有光澤，葉背帶綠蒼
白色，中脈在葉背明顯凸起；葉柄
粗短，被褐色長柔毛。雌雄異株，
傘形花序腋生或節間生，幾無總花
梗及花梗；花被片 6，有稀疏柔
毛；能育雄蕊 9，花藥內向瓣裂，
花絲有稀疏柔毛。果球形，幾無果
梗，成熟時灰藍黑色。花期：七月
至八月。

Lauraceae: Evergreen shrubs or
small trees. Leaves alternate, leathery,
laminae ovate-oblong; apex obtuse or
short acuminate, base cuneiform or
obtuse glossy above, lower surface pale-
green, mid-rib prominently elevated
underneath; petioles stout and short,
brown villose. Dioecious,umbels axillary
or on the internodes, peduncles or
pedicels almost absent; perianth 6-lobed,
sparsely villose; fertile stamens 9, anthers
splitting valvate inwards, filaments
sparsely villose. Fruits globose, almost
sessile, greyish blue-black at maturity.
Flowering from July to August.

絨 毛 潤 楠

Machilus velutina Champ. ex Benth.

別　　名　絨楠、絨毛槙楠、猴高鐵、野枇杷、香膠木。

生長環境　生於山坡溪旁樹林中。

採集加工　藥用根、葉。全年可採，曬乾或鮮用。

性味功能　味苦，性涼。化痰止咳，消腫止痛。

主治用法　支氣管炎，每用葉3至5錢，水煎服。外用治燒燙傷，癰腫，外傷出血，骨折。根或根皮研粉調敷，或鮮品搗爛外敷患處。

方　　例　1.支氣管炎：絨毛潤楠葉（去毛）、桑葉、野菊葉各3錢，水煎服。

2.燒燙傷：絨毛潤楠根或葉適量，研末，麻油調敷，或煎水外洗。

附　　註　本品研粉，加溫開水，即成極黏稠之糊狀物，可作外敷藥的賦形劑，並有消炎止痛的功效。

Habitat　　On slopes, along streams, and in woods.

Preparation　Use roots and leaves. Collect all year round, dry under sun or use fresh.

Properties　Bitter tasting; cool. Expectorant, antitussive; reduces swelling; analgesic.

Indications　Bronchitis. Use leaves 10-15 gm., as decoction. External use in burns and scalds, carbuncles, wound bleeding, fracture. Grind roots or root skin for topical application, or mash fresh herb as poultice.

Prescriptions　1. Bronchitis: Machilus velutina leaves (with hair removed), Morus alba, Chrysanthemum indicum, all using leaves, each 10 gm., as decoction.

2. Burns and scalds: Machilus velutina roots or leaves, finely pulverized and blended with sesame oil as cream or ointment, or boil in water for washing.

Remarks　　The powdered form of this herb when mixed with warm water becomes a very sticky substance which is useful as a mould for topical agents as well as having an anti-inflammatory and analgesic effect.

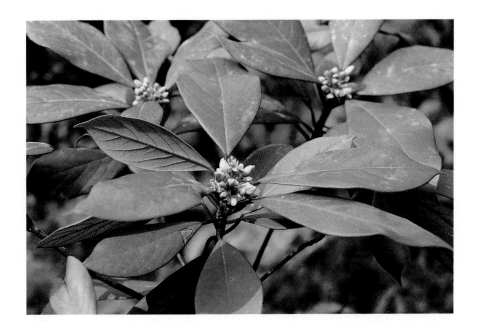

　　樟科、潤楠屬之高大喬木，高可達18米。枝、芽、葉背面、花序均被鏽色密絨毛。葉互生，革質，狹倒卵形或卵狀矩圓形；中脈及側脈均於葉背明顯凸起。圓錐花序短，單獨或數個密集生於小枝頂端；花黃綠色，有香味；花被片6，宿存，反曲，被鏽色絨毛；能育雄蕊9，第三輪雄蕊花絲基部有絨毛，近花絲基部有心形腺體；子房淡紅色。果球形，紫紅色，直徑約4毫米。花期：十一月。

Lauraceae: Large trees, up to 18m high. Branches, buds, lower surface of leaves and infloresences densely covered by pale woolly hairs. Leaves alternate, leathery, narrow obovate or ovate-oblong; both main and lateral veins prominent, elevated on the lower surface. Flowers yellowish green, fragrant, singly or severally in short terminal panicles; perianth segments 6, persistent, recurved, ferruginous tomentose; fertile stamens 9, filaments of stamens in the third whorl tomentose, with cordate glands appearing near the filament bases; ovary pinkish. Fruits globose, purplish-red, about 4mm in diameter. Flowering in November.

萊　菔　子

Raphanus sativus L. var. longipinnatus Bailey

別　　名　蘿蔔、蘿白、蘿卜。

生長環境　多為栽培。

採集加工　藥用種子（萊菔子）為主。種子成熟後，割取全株，曬乾，打下種子，鮮用或炒用。

性味功能　味辛、甘，性平。下氣，化痰，消積滯。

主治用法　1.咳嗽痰多；2.食滯腹脹，便秘；3.痢疾。每用5分至3錢，水煎服。

方　　例　1.慢性氣管炎，咳嗽痰多：萊菔子、蘇子各3錢，白芥子2錢，水煎服。（三子養親湯）

2. 飲食積滯，胃脹口臭：萊菔子、麥芽、穀芽各3錢，雞內金2錢，水煎服。

主要成分　種子含芥子鹼（sinapine）、油（油中含芥子酸、甘油脂及揮發油）。

附　　註　蘿蔔鮮根味辛、甘，性涼。有消積滯，化痰熱，解酒毒功效。適量煎湯或煮食。

Habitat　　　Mostly cultivated.

Preparation　　Use seeds mainly. When seeds ripen, harvest the whole plant and dry under sun, then remove seeds for fresh use or stir fry.

Properties　　Acrid and sweet tasting; neutral. Carminative, liquifies sputum, promotes digestion.

Indications　　1. Productive cough; 2. Indigestion, abdominal distention, constipation; 3. Dysentery. Use 1.5-9 gm., as decoction.

Prescriptions　　1. Chronic bronohitis, productive coughs: Raphanus longipinnatus seeds, Perilla frutescens seeds, 10 gm. each, Brassica alba seeds 6 gm., as decoction.

2. Indigestion, abdominal distention, bad breath: Raphanus longipinnatus seeds, Hordeum vulgare (wheat) germ, Oryza sativa (rice) germ, 10 gm. each, inner lining of chicken gizzards 6 gm., as decoction.

Remarks　　Raphanus longipinnatus fresh root: Acrid and sweet tasting; cool. Promotes digestion, liquifies sputum, and alleviates the effects of alcohol poisoning. Use suitable quantity in soup or in food.

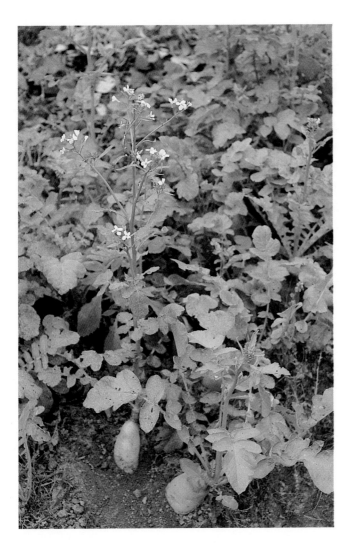

　　十字花科、蘿蔔屬之二年或一
年生草本，高 20 至 100 厘米。全體
粗糙；主根粗壯稍直，肉質，形狀
及大小多變化。基生葉及下部葉呈
大頭羽狀分裂，長 8 至 30 厘米，頂
生裂片卵形，側生裂片 4 至 6 對且向
葉基方向縮小，葉緣有鈍齒，疏生
粗毛；上部葉矩圓形，有鋸齒或近
全緣。總狀花序頂生；花淡紫紅色
或白色。長角果肉質，圓柱形，長
1.5 至 3 厘米，果皮在每粒種子間縮
窄，形成海綿質橫隔，先端漸尖成
喙。種子卵形，微扁，紅褐色。花
期：十一月至翌年三月。

Cruciferae (Brassicaceae): Annual
or biennial herbs, 20-100cm high; rough
throughout; tap root stout, fleshy,
variable in size and shape. Basal leaves
and lower cauline leaves pinnately lobed
and with a large terminal segment, 8-
30cm long, the terminal segment ovate,
lateral segments 4-6 pairs, progressively
decreasing in size towards the base;
margins with obtuse teeth, strigose;
upper cauline leaves oblong, serrate or
subentire. Flowers purplish-white, in
terminal racemes. Siliques fleshy,
cylindrical, 1.5-3cm long, pericarp
constricted between seeds, forming
spongy septa, attenuate at distal end,
forming the beak. Seeds ovoid, slightly
compressed, reddish-brown. Flowering
from November to March of the
following year.

繡 球 花

Hydrangea macrophylla (Thunb.) Seringe

別　　名　八仙花、綉球花、粉團花、紫陽花。

生長環境　栽培於庭園中。

採集加工　藥用葉、花及根。春、夏季採收，曬乾或鮮用。

性味功能　味苦、微辛，性寒。有小毒。清熱解毒，抗瘧。

主治用法　1.瘧疾；2.發熱，心煩；3.咽喉腫痛。每用3至5錢，水煎服。過量易致嘔吐。外用適量煎水洗，治陰囊濕疹。

方　　例　1.瘧疾：繡球花葉3錢，常山2錢，水煎，在瘧疾發作前2小時服。

2. 咽喉腫痛：繡球花根，醋磨汁，含漱。

3. 陰囊濕疹：繡球花，蛇床子，刺莧適量，煎水洗患處。

主要成分　本品含抗瘧生物鹼。花含芸香甙（rutin）乾花中含量超過0.36%。根及其他部分含白瑞香素（daphnetin）的甲基衍生物和傘形花內酯等。

附　　註　本品提取物，對雞瘧疾有顯著療效。

Habitat　　Cultivated in gardens.

Preparation　　Use leaves, flowers, and roots. Collect in spring and summer, dry under sun or use fresh.

Properties　　Bitter and mildly acrid tasting; cold. Slightly toxic. Anti-inflammatory, anti-malarial.

Indications　　1. Malaria; 2. Fever, anxiety; 3. Sore throat. Use 10-15 gm., as decoction. Overdose causes vomiting. For external use in cases of scrotal eczema, boil in water for washing.

Prescriptions　　1. Malaria: Hydrangea macrophylla 10 gm., Dichroa febrifuga 6 gm., as decoction, to be taken two hours prior to malarial attacks.

2. Sore throat: Hydrangea macrophylla roots, add vinegar and grind together, as gargle.

3. Scrotal eczema: Hydrangea macrophylla, Cnidium monnieri fruits, Amaranthus spinosus, in suitable quantities, boil in water to wash affected parts.

Remarks　　The extract of this herb is also useful for malaria of the chickens.

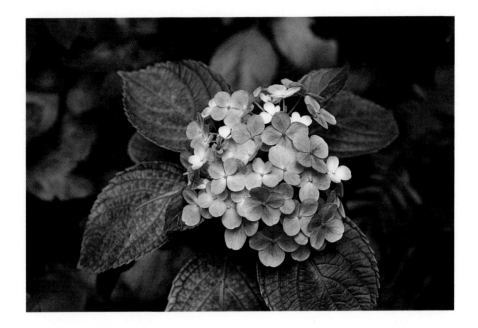

　　虎耳草科、繡球屬之多年生落葉小灌木，高約1米。莖粗壯，皮孔及葉痕明顯，嫩莖綠色。葉對生，密集，節間短；葉片大而稍厚，橢圓形至寬卵形；前端短尖，葉基寬楔形，葉緣具粗鋸齒；葉面鮮綠色，葉背黃綠色。傘房花序頂生，球形，直徑可達20厘米；花梗有柔毛；花極美麗而顯眼，由4至5塊萼片組成，萼片寬卵形至圓形，白色、粉紅色或變為藍色，全部為不育花。花期：五月。

Hydrangeaceae: Small perennial deciduous shrubs, 1m high. Stems stout, lenticels and leaf scars prominent, stems green when young. Leaves opposite, dense, internodes short; laminae large and thick, elliptic to broad ovate; apex abruptly acute, base broad cuneate; margins serrate; green above, yellowish green beneath. Flowers all sterile, showy, coloured white, pink or becoming blue, consisting of 4-5 large sepals, shaped broad ovate to orbicular, and forming globular terminal corymbs up to 20cm in diameter; pedicels pilose. Flowering in May.

春花木（車輪梅）

Rhaphiolepis indica (L.) Lindl.

別　　名　春花、石斑木、石桂、雷公樹。

生長環境　生於向陽山坡、路邊灌木叢中。

採集加工　藥用根、葉。全年可採，曬乾或鮮用。

性味功能　味微苦，性涼。消腫解毒。

主治用法　1.跌打損傷；2.關節炎。每用根3至5錢，水煎服。外用治潰瘍紅腫，瘡癤，骨髓炎。鮮葉適量搗敷，或乾葉研粉外敷。

方　　例　1.跌打損傷：春花木根3錢，水煎服；外用鮮葉搗敷患處。

2. 足踝關節陳舊傷作痛：春花木根3斤，切片，加川牛膝4兩，用燒酒10斤浸一個月後，去渣取酒，每日飯前適量服。

主要成分　樹皮含鞣質。

Habitat	On sunny slopes and in roadside thickets.
Preparation	Use roots and leaves. Collect all year round. Dry under sun or use fresh.
Properties	Slightly bitter tasting; cool. Anti-swelling, anti-inflammatory.
Indications	1. Traumatic injury; 2. Arthritis. Use roots 10-15 gm., as decoction. External use in ulcers, erythematous ulcer, furunculosis, osteomyelitis. Mash fresh leaves for poultice, or grind dry leaves for external application.
Prescriptions	1. Traumatic injury: Rhaphiolepis indica roots 10 gm., as decoction. For external use, mash fresh leaves for topical application.

2. Ankle joint chronic pain: Rhaphiolepis indica 3 catties (1.8 kg.), slice, add Achyranthes bidentata 120 gm., steep in 10 catties of wine for one month, drain and take wine once daily before meal.

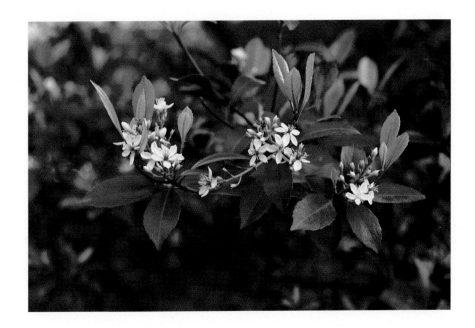

　　薔薇科、車輪梅屬之常綠直立灌木。小枝條初時被褐色絨毛，後脫落。葉互生，革質，厚而光亮，葉形有卵形、矩圓形、披針形等，葉基狹而成一短柄，葉緣有小鋸齒。稍稠密的圓錐花序或總狀花序頂生，總花梗及花梗密生鏽色絨毛；花白色而帶粉紅，鮮艷奪目，直徑約1厘米；苞片膜質；萼管無毛或被絨毛，裂片長尖形；花瓣約與萼片等長。梨果球形，紫黑色，可食。花期：三月。

Rosaceae: Erect evergreen shrubs. Young branches with brown woolly hairs which subsequently fall off. Leaves alternate, leathery, thick and glossy; laminae ovate, oblong or lanceolate; base narrowed to form a short stalk, margins serrulate. Flowers showy, white, tinged pink, 1cm in diameter, in terminal panicles or racemes, peduncles and pedicels densely tomentose, ferruginous; bracts membranous; calyx tubular, pilose or glabrous, lobes acuminate; petals and sepals about equal in length. Pomes globose, purplish black, edible. Flowering in March.

紅 葉 藤

Rourea microphylla (Hook. et Arn.) Planch.

別　　名　牛見愁、牛栓藤、荔枝藤、霸王藤。

生長環境　生於山地、路旁、灌木叢中。

採集加工　藥用根、葉。全年可採，切段，鮮用或曬乾備用。

性味功能　味微辛、甘，性溫。活血通經，止血止痛。

主治用法　經閉，每用根3至5錢，水煎服。小兒熱毒瘡，跌打損傷腫痛，外傷出血，鮮葉搗爛外敷，或煎水洗患處。

主要成分　根、莖、樹皮含鞣質。

Habitat　　On hills, along roadside and in thickets.

Preparation　　Use roots and leaves. Collect all year round. Cut into segments, use fresh or dry under sun.

Properties　　Slightly acrid and sweet tasting; warm. Promotes circulation, regulates menstruation; haemostatic, analgesic.

Indications　　Amenorrhea, use roots 10-15 gm., as decoction. Pyodermas in children, traumatic injury and wound bleeding, mash fresh leaves and apply to lesion; may also boil in water and wash affected parts.

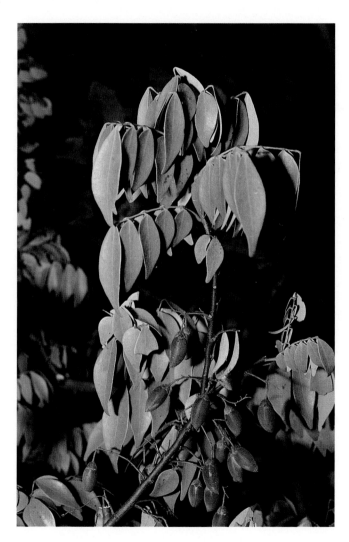

　　牛栓藤科、紅葉藤屬之藤狀灌木，高不逾２米。奇數羽狀複葉，小葉卵形至卵狀矩圓形；葉基偏斜；上表面光亮。總狀花序，叢生於葉腋，總花梗及花梗均纖弱；花白色，有香氣，長５至７毫米；萼片５，三角形，宿存，開花後萼片長度較開花前長；花瓣５；雄蕊１０，長短不等，花絲基部合生；心皮５，離生，常只有１個發育。蓇葖果橙黃色，略彎曲。種子１枚，外有膜質假種皮。花期：三月至九月。

Connaraceae: Climbing shrubs, not exceeding 2m high. Leaves odd-pinnate, leaflets ovate to ovate-oblong; base oblique; glossy above. Flowers white, fragrant, 5-7mm long, in clustering axillary racemes; both peduncles and pedicels delicate;sepals 5, deltoid, persistent, sepals lengthening at bloom; petals 5; stamens 10, of various lengths, filament bases connate; carpels 5, distinct, frequently only one developing. Follicles orange, slightly curved. Seed 1, aril membranous. Flowering from March to September.

華 南 雲 實

Caesalpinia nuga (L.) Ait.

別　　名　假老虎簕、虎耳藤、見血飛、南天藤。

生長環境　生於山地、樹林中。

採集加工　藥用根為主。秋、冬採挖，曬乾。

性味功能　味甘、淡，性微寒。清熱利尿，袪風濕。種子：止咳。

主治用法　1. 熱淋（尿道感染）；2. 風濕痹痛。每用 3 至 4 錢，水煎服。外用治外傷腫痛，筋骨痛，瘡癤。

方　　例　瘡癤腫毒：華南雲實根或葉，雞屎藤適量，煎水洗患處。

附　　註　印度用華南雲實根為利尿劑，治膀胱結石；莖汁內服治眼病；葉粉末為婦人產後子宮強壯劑。

Habitat　　　In mountainous area and in woods.

Preparation　Use roots mainly. Collect in autumn and winter, dry under sun.

Properties　Sweet and bland tasting; slightly cold. Anti-inflammatory, diuretic, anti-rheumatic. Seeds: antitussive.

Indications　1. Urinary tract infection; 2. Rheumatism. Use 10-12 gm., as decoction. External use in wounds and swelling, joint pains, furunculosis.

Prescription　Furunculosis: Caesalpinia nuga roots or leaves and Paederia scandens in sufficient amounts, boil in water for washing.

Remarks　　In India, the roots of this herb are used as a diuretic in cases of bladder stones. The juice extract of the stem is used for curing eye diseases. The ground powder from leaves is used as postpartum uterine tonic.

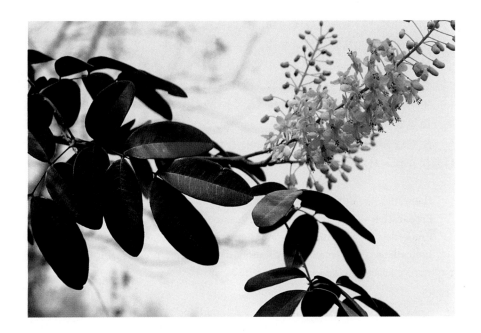

　　豆科、雲實屬之藤本。莖有倒鈎刺，嫩莖被紅棕色絨毛。2回羽狀複羽，羽片4至10塊，小葉革質，長橢圓形，葉尖端鈍或微缺。圓錐花序頂生或腋生，花數目多；萼筒闊倒圓錐形；花瓣5，黃色；雄蕊10，分離，花絲下部被疏柔毛；子房有短柄。莢果棕黑色，革質，闊短圓形，偏斜，頂端急尖，先端有喙，果身扁，長3.5至4厘米，寬2至2.5厘米。種子1枚。花期：三月至四月。

Leguminoceae: Vines, stems barbed, young stems reddish brown tomentose. Leaves bipinnate, pinnae 4-10; leaflets leathery, oblong; apex obtuse or emarginate. Flowers numerous, yellow, in terminal or axillary panicles; calyx tube broad obconic; petals 5; stamens 10, distinct, filaments sparsely pubescent at base; ovary with short stalk. Pods brownish black, leathery, broad oblong, oblique, apex acute and beaked, compressed, 3.5-4cm long by 2-2.5cm wide. Seed 1. Flowering from March to April.

有 翅 決 明

Cassia alata L.

別　　名　對葉豆、翅莢決明、非洲木通。

生長環境　栽培於庭園或路旁。

採集加工　藥用葉為主。全年可採，多為鮮用。

性味功能　味辛，性溫。解毒，瀉下，殺蟲。

主治用法　1.神經性皮炎，牛皮癬；2.濕疹，皮膚瘙癢；3.瘡癤腫瘍。外用鮮葉搗汁搽患處。

主要成分　葉含蒽醌類、黃酮類化合物，已知有大黃酸（rhein）。果實亦含蒽醌類化合物。故有瀉下，抗菌作用。

Habitat　　　Cultivated in gardens and by curbside.

Preparation　Use leaves. Collect all year round, use fresh.

Properties　Acrid tasting; warm. Anti-inflammatory, laxative, vermifuge.

Indications　1. Neurodermatitis, psoriasis; 2. Eczema, pruritus; 3. Pyoderma. For external use, squeeze juice from leaves and apply to lesion.

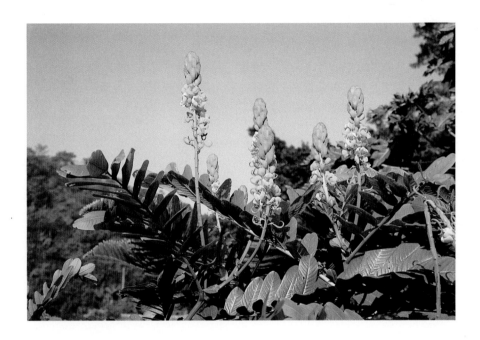

　　豆科、決明屬之灌木至小喬木。偶數羽狀複葉，幾近無葉柄，長30至60厘米；小葉5至12對，硬革質，矩圓形；葉先端細尖；葉基闊圓形，左右略不對稱，一邊偏大；葉軸兩邊有狹翅。總狀花序生於莖頂，長15至30厘米；苞片大，三角形，膜質，早落；花黃色，花瓣上之脈多而明顯；各雄蕊極不相等。莢果長舌狀，膜質，熟時開裂，豆莢每果瓣之中央均有由頂縱貫至基部之闊翅。花期：六月至九月。

Leguminoceae: Shrubs or small trees. Leaves even-pinnate, nearly sessile, 30-60cm long; leaflets 5-12 pairs, firm leathery, oblong; apex apiculate, base broad rounded, slightly asymmetrical; rachis with narrow wings on either side. Flowers yellow, in terminal racemes 15-30cm long; bracts large, deltoid, membranous, caducous; veins on petals numerous and prominent; stamens extremely unequal. Pods in the shape of long tongues, membranous, possessing a wing which runs the whole length of the pod at the middle of each side, dehiscent at maturity. Flowering from June to September.

黃　槐

Cassia surattensis Burm. f.

生長環境　栽培於庭園或路旁。

採集加工　藥用葉、花、果。全年可採，曬乾或鮮用。

性味功能　味苦，性涼。葉：清熱，止咳，瀉下。花、果：清熱，止血。

主治用法　葉：咽喉腫痛，風熱咳嗽，便秘。每用 1 至 3 錢，水煎服，或泡茶服。花、果：痔瘡出血。每用 2 至 3 錢，水煎服。

Habitat　　　Cultivated in gardens or by roadside.

Preparation　　Use leaves, flowers, fruits (seed pods). Collect all year round, dry under sun or use fresh.

Properties　　Bitter tasting; cool. Leaves: anti-inflammatory, antitussive, purgative. Flowers and fruits: anti-inflammatory, haemostatic.

Indications　　Leaves: dry coughs, sore throat, constipation. Use 3-10 gm., as decoction or as tea. Flowers and fruits: Bleeding haemorrhoids. Use 5-10 gm., as decoction.

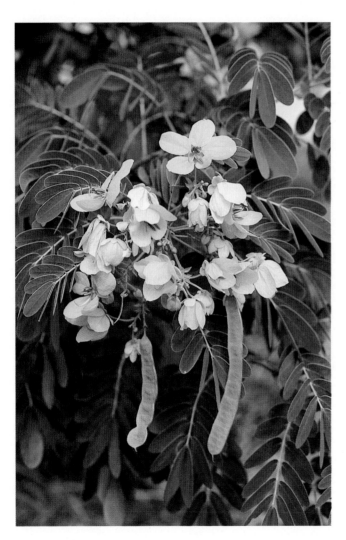

　　豆科、決明屬之小喬木。偶數羽狀複葉，小葉14至18片，長橢圓形或卵形；葉先端圓而微凹，葉基圓而常偏斜；葉背面粉綠色，被短毛；葉柄及最後之2至3對小葉之葉軸上有2或3枚棍棒狀腺體。總狀花序生於枝條上部之葉腋處；花黃色或深黃色；雄蕊10，下方之2至3枚雄蕊之花藥較大；子房有毛。莢果長條形，長7至10厘米，種子間微縊成節莢，果先端有喙。花期：九月至十二月。

Leguminoceae: Small trees. Leaves even-pinnate, pinnae 14-18, oblong or ovate; apex rounded, emarginate; base rounded or oblique; light green beneath, pilose; 2 or 3 clavate glands on the petioles and on the last two to three pairs of rachis. Flowers yellow or deep yellow, in axillary racemes on upper branches; stamens 10, the lower two or three with larger anthers; ovary hairy. Pods linear, 7-10cm long, apex beaked, pods slightly constricted between seeds. Flowering from September to December.

台 灣 相 思

Acacia confusa Merr.

別　　名　相思樹。

生長環境　栽培於山野路邊。在香港廣泛栽種以穩固山坡。

採集加工　藥用枝、葉。全年可採，多為鮮用。

性味功能　味甘、淡，性平。去腐生肌。

主治用法　多外用於跌打損傷，瘡瘍。外用適量，煎水洗患處，有消腫及促進肉芽生長作用。

方　　例　跌打損傷：台灣相思嫩芽絞汁，加酒、水少許冲服。

主要成分　樹皮含鞣質 15%。種子含有毒成分。

附　　註　種子有毒，誤食會引起腹痛、頭痛、噁心、嘔吐。

Habitat　　　Cultivated in fields and on roadside. Widely planted in Hong Kong to stabilize slopes.

Preparation　　Use branches and leaves. Collect all year round, use fresh.

Properties　　Sweet and bland tasting; neutral. Promotes granulation healing.

Indications　　External use in traumatic injury, wounds. Boil herb in water for washing. Reduces swelling and promotes healing.

Prescription　　Traumatic injury: Acacia confusa shoots extract, blend with wine and water for consumption.

Remarks　　The seeds are poisonous. Ingestion causes headache, stomachache, nausea, and vomiting.

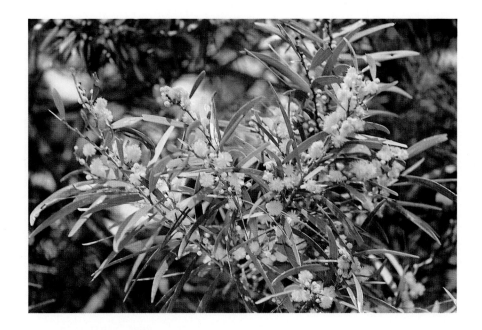

　　豆科、金合歡屬之常綠喬木，優美，高可達 15 米，分枝多，幼莖略下垂。見到之"葉"是由葉柄變態而成，稱"葉狀柄"，互生，革質，披針鐮形，兩端尖狹，平行葉脈3至5條。絨球狀之頭狀花序多數，微香，美麗，黃色，6至8毫米大，單個或兩個腋生；花瓣2毫米長；雄蕊多數；子房有毛；莢果扁，幼時有柔毛，莢乾時深褐色，節莢狀。種子7至8粒，扁橢圓形。花期：四月至五月。

　　Leguminoceae: Graceful evergreen trees, up to 15m high, many branches, young ones slightly drooping. Petioles having appearance of leaves, called "phyllodes", alternate, leathery, lanceolate falcate, attenuate at both ends, 3-5 parallel veins. Yellow pom-pon flowers numerous, small, scented, beautiful, globose head 6-8mm across, 1 or 2 heads in a leaf axil; petals 2mm long; stamens numerous; ovary hairy. Pods flattened, pilose when young, dark brown when dried, constricted between seeds. Seeds 7-8, compressed elliptic. Flowering from April to May.

響 鈴 豆

Crotalaria albida Heyne ex Roth

別　　名　黃花地丁、馬口鈴、小響鈴、響鈴草。

生長環境　生於山坡草叢、海邊荒地。

採集加工　藥用全草。夏、秋季採收，切段，曬乾。

性味功能　味苦、辛，性涼。清熱解毒，止咳平喘。

主治用法　1.尿道炎，膀胱炎；2. 支氣管炎，久咳痰喘；3. 胃腸炎，肝炎；4.瘧疾。每用3至5錢，水煎服。外用治癰瘡腫毒，乳腺炎，腮腺炎，淋巴腺炎，鮮葉適量搗爛外敷患處。

方　　例　尿道炎，膀胱炎：響鈴豆1 至 1.5 兩，水煎服，白酒為引。曾治療100 餘例，效果良好。

主要成分　種子含野百合鹼、響鈴豆鹼（croalbidine）。

Habitat　　In bushes on slopes and along seaside.

Preparation　　Use whole herb. Collect in summer and autumn, cut into segments, dry under sun.

Properties　　Bitter and acrid tasting; cool. Anti-inflammatory, antitussive, anti-asthmatic.

Indications　　1. Urinary tract infection, cystitis; 2. Bronchitis, prolonged cough, wheezing; 3. Gastroenteritis, hepatitis; 4. Malaria. Use 10-15 gm., as decoction. External use in furuncles, carbuncles, mastitis, parotitis, lymphadenitis. Mash fresh leaves for topical application.

Prescription　　Urinary tract infection, cystitis: Crotalaria albida 30-45 gm., as decoction, to take with wine. More than 100 cases have been treated with good results.

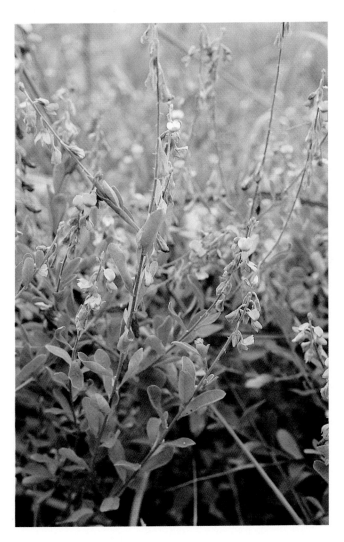

　　豆科、野百合屬之灌木狀草本，高 30 至 150 厘米。被白色柔毛。葉互生，倒卵狀披針形至倒披針形；葉頂端鈍圓，有小凸尖，葉基狹楔形；葉面光滑，葉底生疏柔毛；托葉細小。總狀花序頂生或腋生；小苞片着生於花萼基部；花萼深裂，上面2萼齒橢圓形，下面3萼齒披針形，均有短柔毛；花冠黃色，稍長於萼。莢果圓柱形，膨脹，表面光滑，有種子6至12粒。花期：四月至十月。

Leguminoceae: Subshrubs or herbs, 30-150 cm high, white pilose. Leaves alternate, obovate-lanceolate to oblanceolate; apex obtuse-apiculate, base narrow cuneate; glabrous above, sparsely pilose beneath; stipules minute. Flowers in terminal or axillary racemes; calyx bearing bracteoles at the base, deeply lobed, upper two teeth elliptic, lower three lanceolate, all teeth pilose; corolla yellow, slightly longer than calyx. Pods cylindrical, swelling, glabrous. Seeds 6-12. Flowering from April to October.

旱 金 蓮

Tropaeolum majus L.

別　　名　旱蓮花、金蓮花。

生長環境　多栽培於庭園。

採集加工　藥用全草。秋、冬採收，多鮮用。

性味功能　味辛、酸，性涼。清熱解毒。

主治用法　1. 眼結膜炎，目赤腫痛；2. 癰癤腫毒；3. 跌打損傷。多作外用，鮮品適量搗敷患處。

方　　例　1. 眼結膜炎：金蓮花、野菊花各適量，搗爛敷眼眶周圍。

2. 癰癤腫毒：金蓮花、霧水葛、木芙蓉各適量，搗爛敷患處。

主要成分　種子含揮發成分異硫氰酸苄脂（benzyl isothiocyanate）等；莖葉含異槲皮甙（isoquercitroside）等；花含山奈酚葡萄糖甙（kaempferol glucoside）等。

Habitat　　　Mostly cultivated in gardens.

Preparation　　Use whole herb. Collect in autumn and winter, use fresh.

Properties　　Acrid, sour tasting; cool. Anti-inflammatory.

Indications　　1. Conjunctivitis, sore eyes; 2. furuncles and carbuncles; 3. Traumatic injury. Mostly used externally. Mash fresh herb for local application.

Prescriptions　　1. Conjunctivitis: Tropaeolum majus, Chrysanthemum indicum flowers, each in suitable amount, mash and apply in periorbital area.

2. Furuncles and carbuncles: Tropaeolum majus, Pouzolzia zeylanica, Hibiscus mutabilis leaves in suitable amounts, mash and apply to lesion.

Remarks　　　The seeds contain benzyl isothiocyanate; stem and leaves contain isoquercitroside; flowers contain kaempferol glucoside.

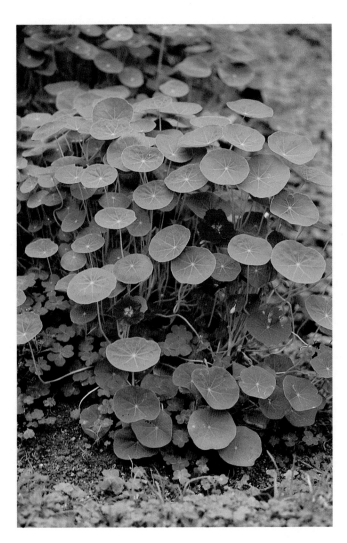

　　旱金蓮科、旱金蓮屬之一年生攀援狀肉質草本，全株光滑。葉互生，近圓形，長約10厘米；有主脈9條，自中央放射狀發出；葉緣有波狀鈍角；葉柄長，盾狀着生於葉片之近中央處。花單生於葉腋，有長柄；花黃色或橘紅色；萼片5片，基部合生，其中1片延長成一長距；花瓣5片，大小不等，上面2瓣常較大，花瓣基部狹窄成爪形；雄蕊8枚，不等長；柱頭3裂，綫形。核果。花期：春季至夏季。

Tropaeolaceae: Annual creeping succulent herbs, glabrous. Leaves peltate, alternate, suborbicular, 10cm long; main veins 9, radiating from the centre of the leaf; margin undulate with obtuse protrusions; petioles long, joining the lamina near its centre. Flowers yellowish or orange-red, solitary, axillary, pedicels long; sepals 5, connate at the base, one of which spur-like; petals 5, of various sizes, upper two larger, with narrow unguiculate base; stamens 8, of unequal length; stigma trifid, linear. Drupes. Flowering from spring to summer.

檸　　檬

Citrus limonia Osbeck

別　　名　　黎檬、藥果、夢子。

生長環境　　多為栽培。

採集加工　　藥用果、根、葉。根、葉全年可採，果秋、冬季採。

性味功能　　果：味酸、甘，性平。生津健胃，化痰止咳。根：味辛、苦，性溫。行氣止痛，止咳平喘。葉：味辛、甘，性溫。化痰止咳，開胃。

主治用法　　果：1.食慾不振；2.缺乏維他命C；3.支氣管炎，百日咳；4.中暑煩渴。根：1.胃痛；2.疝氣痛，睪丸炎；3.咳嗽，支氣管哮喘。葉：1.咳喘；2.腹脹，腹瀉。每用鮮果5錢至1兩，根1至2兩，葉3至5錢，水煎服。

方　　例　　鮮檸檬汁：鮮檸檬2個，切開，搾汁。冰糖4兩，水250毫升，煮溶，待冷後，倒入檸檬汁，冷開水加至1公升，放冰箱內。有開胃解渴功效。

主要成分　　檸檬果汁中含枸櫞酸、半乳糖醛酸、維他命A、B、C等。果皮含揮發油檸檬烯、橙皮甙等。葉及木部含揮發油牻牛兒酸等。

Habitat　　Mostly cultivated, as lemon.

Preparation　　Use fruits, roots and leaves. Roots and leaves can be collected all year round. Fruits are collected in autumn and winter.

Properties　　Fruit: Sour and sweet tasting; neutral. Promotes salivary secretion; stomachic, expectorant, antitussive. Roots: Acrid and bitter tasting; warm. Promote circulation; analgesic, antitussive, anti-asthmatic. Leaves: Acrid and sweet tasting; warm. Antitussive, expectorant; stimulate appetite.

Indications　　Fruit: 1. Anorexia; 2. Vitamin C deficiency; 3. Bronchiolitis; 4. Heat stroke. Roots: 1. Epigastric pain; 2. Hernial pain, orchitis; 3. Coughs, bronchial asthma. Leaves: 1. Asthma; 2. Bloatedness, diarrhea. Use fresh fruit 15-30 gm., roots 30-60 gm., leaves 10-15 gm., as decoction.

Prescription　　Fresh lemon juice, with rock sugar, diluted with water, has appetizing and thirst quenching effects.

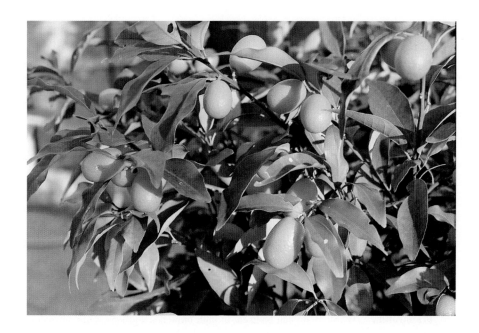

　　芸香科、金橘屬之常綠灌木或小喬木，分枝多。葉互生，披針形至矩圓形，紙質至革質，全緣或具不明顯之細鋸齒；葉面深綠色，光亮，葉背青綠色，有散生腺點，葉有香氣；葉柄有狹翅，與葉片連接處有關節。單花或2至3朵集生於葉腋；花白色，芳香；萼片及花瓣均 5 片；雄蕊 20 至 25 ，長短不一，不同程度的合生成若干束。果矩圓形或卵形，金黃色，皮多腺點，有香味。花期：十一月至翌年二月。

Rutaceae: Evergreen shrubs or small trees, branches numerous. Leaves alternate, aromatic, lanceolate to orbicular-oblong, texture papery to leathery, margins entire or inconspicuously serrulate; glossy dark green above, green beneath, with scattered glands; petioles with narrow wings, connecting to the blades through joints. Flowers white, fragrant, solitary or 2-3 appearing in leaf axils; sepals 5, petals 5; stamens 20-25, of various lengths, grouped variously into several bundles. Fruits oblong or oval, golden, numerous glands on the rind, fragrant. Flowering from November to February of the following year.

苦　木

Picrasma quassioides (D. Don) Benn.

別　　名　苦樹、苦樹皮、苦肥木、山苦楝、山熊膽。

生長環境　生於山坡、路邊潮濕處。

採集加工　藥用全株，以枝、葉較常用。全年可採，曬乾。

性味功能　味苦，性寒。有小毒。清熱解毒。

主治用法　1. 感冒；2. 急性扁桃體炎，咽喉炎；3. 腸炎，菌痢。每用枝1錢至1錢5分，葉3分至1錢，水煎服。孕婦忌服。外用治急性化膿性感染，濕疹，毒蛇咬傷。

方　　例　1. 急性化膿性感染：苦木2份，金櫻根1份。水煎三次，合併過濾後，濃縮成膏，外敷。

2. 菌痢：苦木研粉，每次1至3克，每日服3至4次。

主要成分　樹幹含苦木苦素（quassin）、異苦木素（picrasmin）等。

附　　註　本品有毒部位在根皮、樹皮及葉。食多量會引起咽喉、胃部疼痛，嘔吐、瀉下，眩暈、抽搐，嚴重者休克。

Habitat　　On damp soil on slopes and roadside.

Preparation　　Whole plant can be used, though branches and leaves are more commonly used. Collect all year round, dry under sun.

Properties　　Bitter tasting; cold. Slightly toxic. Anti-inflammatory.

Indications　　1. Influenza; 2. Acute tonsillitis, pharyngitis; 3. Enteritis, bacillary dysentery. Use branches 3-4.5 gm., leaves 1-3 gm., as decoction. Contraindicated in pregnancy. External use in acute pyogenous infection, eczema, snake bites.

Prescriptions　　1. Acute pyogenous infection: Two parts of Picrasma quassioides, one part of Rosa laevigata roots, brew in water three times, filter, and concentrate to become an ointment for topical use.

2. Bacillary dysentery: Picrasma quassioides, grind into powder, take 1-3 gm. orally 3 to 4 times a day.

Remarks　　The trunk contains quassin and picrasmin. The root skin, bark, and leaves are toxic. Excessive intake can cause sorethroat, gastric pain, vomiting, dizziness, convulsion, and shock.

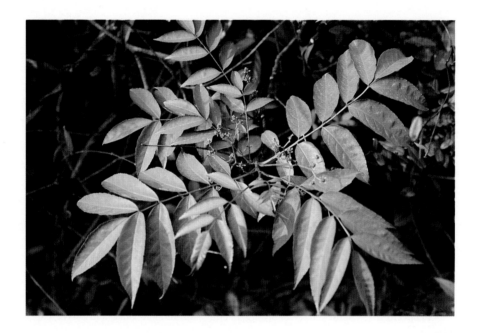

苦木科、苦木屬之灌木或小喬木，高可達10米。嫩莖上有黃色皮孔。奇數羽狀複葉互生，長 20 至 30 厘米；小葉 9 至 15，卵形至矩圓狀卵形，葉頂端銳尖至短漸尖，葉基部寬楔形而偏斜，葉緣具鋸齒。聚傘花序腋生，總花梗長達12厘米，被柔毛。花雜性異株，黃綠色；萼片卵形，被毛；花瓣 4 至 5 片，倒卵形；雄蕊 4 至 5 枚，着生於花盤基部。核果倒卵形，藍至紅色，花萼宿存。花期：四月至五月。

Simaroubaceae: Shrubs or small trees, up to 10m high. Stems with yellowish lenticels when young. Leaves imparipinnate, alternate, 20-30cm long; pinnae 9-15, ovate to oblong-ovate, apex acute to short-acuminate, base broad cuneate, oblique, margins serrate. Flowers yellowish-green, polygamous, cymes axillary, peduncles to 12cm long, pilose; petals 4-5, obovate; stamens 4-5, borne on the base of the floral disc. Drupes obovate, blue to red, sepals persistent. Flowering from April to May.

大 金 牛 草
Polygala glomerata Lour.

別　　名　大金草、大金不換、金不換、肥兒草、華南遠志。

生長環境　生於山坡、路旁草叢中。

採集加工　藥用全草。夏、秋採集，曬乾或鮮用。

性味功能　味辛、甘，性平。清熱解毒，祛痰止咳，活血散瘀。

主治用法　1. 咳嗽，咯血，支氣管炎；2. 急性結膜炎，咽炎；3. 肝炎，黃疸；4. 小兒疳積。每用5錢至1兩，水煎服。外用治瘡癤，跌打損傷，蛇咬傷，鮮品適量搗敷患處。

方　　例　1. 風熱咳嗽：大金牛草、三加皮根各1兩，牛大力、毛鵝桐各5錢，水煎服。

2. 咯血：鮮大金牛草1兩，麥冬3錢，冰糖適量，水煎服。

主要成分　全草含蘇漆內酯（suchilactone）、漆蘇內酯（chisulactone）及賽菊芋色素（helioxanthin）等。

Habitat　　On slopes and among roadside bushes.

Preparation　　Use whole herb. Collect in summer and autumn, dry under sun or use fresh.

Properties　　Acrid and sweet tasting; neutral. Anti-inflammatory, antitussive, expectorant; promotes circulation, resorbs bruises.

Indications　　1. Coughs, haemoptysis, bronchitis; 2. Acute conjunctivitis, pharyngitis; 3. Hepatitis, jaundice; 4. Infantile malabsorption. Use 15-30 gm., as decoction. External use in furunculosis, traumatic injury, snake bites. Mash fresh herb for use as poultice.

Prescriptions　　1. Coughs: Polygala glomerata, Acanthopanax trifoliatus root, 30 gm. each, Millettia speciosa root and Clerodendrum petasites root, 15 gm. each, as decoction.

2. Haemoptysis: Fresh Polygala glomerata 30 gm., Ophiopogon japonica 10 gm., add rock sugar and brew as decoction.

Remarks　　The whole herb contains suchilactone, chisulactone and helioxanthin.

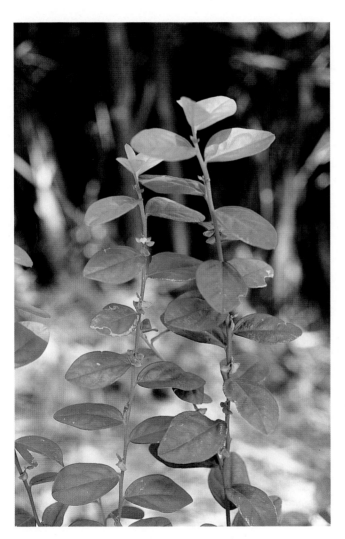

　　遠志科、遠志屬之一年生直立草本，高10至40厘米。葉互生，葉質稍厚，橢圓形至矩圓狀披針形。短小之總狀花序腋生或腋外生，具數朵淡黃色之小花；萼片宿存，外輪3片，內輪2片為花瓣狀；花瓣3片，中間龍骨瓣背面頂有雞冠狀附屬物，兩側花瓣與花絲鞘在基部貼生；雄蕊8，花絲下部合生成鞘。蒴果近倒心形，邊緣有睫毛。種子2，除假種皮外，密被絹狀毛。花期：九月。

Polygalaceae: Annual erect herbs, 10-40cm high. Leaves alternate, lamina thick, ovate to oblong-lanceolate. Flowers light yellow, small, short racemes axillary or exo-axillary; sepals persistent, outer whorl 3, inner whorl petaloid 2; petals 3, with cristate appendage at top of the dorsal side of the keel, the bases of two lateral petals and filament sheath connate; stamens 8, bases fused to form a sheath. Capsules obcordate, margins with ciliate hairs. Seeds 2, densely sericeus except the aril. Flowering in September.

土　蜜　樹

Bridelia tomentosa Bl.

別　　名　土知母、夾骨木、逼迫子、補鍋樹、補腦根。

生長環境　生於山坡、路旁灌木叢中。

採集加工　藥用根皮、莖、葉。全年可採，切段曬乾。

性味功能　味淡、微苦，性平。安神調經，清熱解毒。

主治用法　1. 神經衰弱；2. 精神分裂症；3. 月經不調；4. 犬咬傷。每用根皮 5
錢至 1 兩，水煎服。外用治瘡癤腫毒，跌打損傷，外傷出血，鮮葉搗爛外敷。

方　　例　犬咬傷：土蜜樹莖、葉 1 至 2 兩，水煎服。

主要成分　葉含黃酮貳、無羈萜、無羈萜烷 - 3β - 醇（friedelan - 3β - ol）、豆甾
醇、β - 谷甾醇等。

Habitat　　On slopes and among roadside bushes.

Preparation　　Use the root skin, stem, and leaves. Collect all year round, cut into segments, dry under sun.

Properties　　Bland and slightly bitter tasting; neutral. Sedative; regulates menses; anti-inflammatory.

Indications　　1. Neurasthenia; 2. Schizophrenia, irregular menses; 4. Dog bites. Use root skin 15-30 gm., as decoction. External use in pyodermas, traumatic injury, wound bleeding. Mash fresh herb and apply to lesion.

Prescription　　Dog bites: Stem and leaves of Bridelia tomentosa 30-60 gm., as decoction.

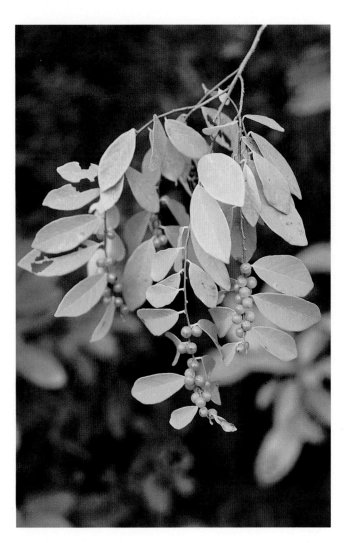

大戟科、土蜜樹屬之直立灌木，高1至5米。幼莖纖細，密被鏽色短柔毛。葉互生，長橢圓形至倒卵狀矩圓形，紙質；葉底被密長柔毛；葉尖端銳尖或鈍；葉柄被密而短之鏽色柔毛；托葉條狀披針形。花細小，單性，雌雄同株，數朵簇生於葉腋；花瓣5，萼片5；雄花花盤杯狀，雄蕊5；雌花花盤環狀，花柱2。核果卵狀球形，長5至7毫米，寬約5毫米。花期：四月。

Euphorbiaceae: Annual shrubs, erect, 1-5m high. Young stems slender, densely ferrugineous pilose. Leaves alternate, elliptic to obovate-oblong, papery; lower surface densely villose; apex acute to obtuse; stipules linear-lanceolate. Flowers small, unisexual, monoecious, several flowers fasciculate on the axils; petals 5; sepals 5; staminate (male flower) disc cup-like, stamens 5; pistillate (female flower) disc annular, styles 2. Drupes ovate-globose, 5-7mm long, 5mm wide. Flowering in April.

艾 膠 樹

Glochidion lanceolarium (Roxb.) Voigt

別　　名　大葉算盤子、山疳黃。

生長環境　生於向陽的山坡或村邊。

採集加工　藥用根、莖、葉。全年可採，曬乾用。

性味功能　清熱解毒。

主治用法　根：黃疸。莖、葉：口腔炎，牙齦炎，跌打外傷。每用5錢至1兩，水煎服。外用適量，鮮葉搗敷患處。

主要成分　莖含無羈萜、3β-無羈萜醇（friedelan-3-01）、算盤子酮、算盤子酮醇（glochidonol）、算盤子二醇等。葉含β-谷甾醇及豆甾醇等。

Habitat	On sunny slopes or village edges.
Preparation	Use root, stems, leaves. Collect all year round, dry under sun.
Properties	Anti-inflammatory.
Indications	Root: Jaundice. Stems and leaves: Stomatitis, gum inflammation, traumatic injury. Use 15-30 gm., as decoction. For external use, mash fresh herb as poultice.

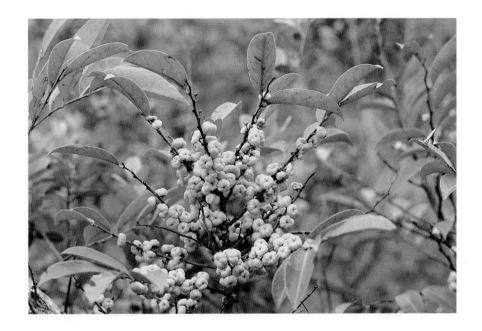

　　大戟科、算盤子屬之灌木。嫩枝各節間順序向左右彎曲生長，無毛。葉互生，革質，橢圓形至長圓形，無毛；托葉披針形。雌雄同株異花，花簇生於葉腋，無花瓣；雄花萼片6，雄蕊5至6；雌花萼片6，子房7至8室。蒴果扁球形，頂端深凹陷，具6至8條縱溝。花期：五月至六月。

　　Euphorbiaceae: Shrubs. Young branches zigzag, glabrous. Leaves alternate, leathery, elliptic to oblong, glabrous; stipules lanceolate. Flowers unisexual, monoecious, flowers in axillary clusters, without petals; male flowers with 6 sepals, stamens 5-6; female flowers with 6 sepals, ovary with 7-8 chambers. Capsules compressed globose, tip deeply depressed, longitudinal furrows 6-8. Flowering from May to June.

粗　糠　柴

Mallotus philippinensis (Lam.) Muell.-Arg.

別　　名　呂宋揪毛、香檀、香桂樹、六檢子、雞尾樹。

生長環境　生於溪邊和山谷的疏林中。

採集加工　藥用根、葉、果毛。根、葉全年可採。果毛於果實成熟時採下，入布袋中，磨擦搓揉，收集擦落毛茸，揀去果實，乾燥即可。

性味功能　根：味微苦、澀，性涼。清熱利濕。果毛（腺體粉，又名呂宋揪莢粉）：味淡，性平。有毒。驅蟲，瀉下。

主治用法　根：1. 急、慢性痢疾；2. 咽喉腫痛。每用3錢，水煎服。果毛：驅除縧蟲、蛔蟲、蟯蟲，並有瀉下作用。每用1至2錢，研末內服。葉：外用於瘡瘍潰爛，外傷出血。

方　　例　瘡瘍潰爛久不收口：粗糠柴葉煎水外洗，並用葉研粉撒敷患處。

主要成分　含樹脂65-73%及蠟質2%。樹脂中含卡馬拉素及異卡馬拉素。

附　　註　粗糠柴的果及葉下暗紅色粉末狀小點均有毒。中毒主要症狀為噁心、嘔吐及嚴重腹瀉。

Habitat　　　Along creeks and in woods in valleys.

Preparation　　Use roots, leaves, and the hair of the fruit. Collect leaves and roots all year round. When fruits are ripe, collect into a sack, rub and knead to detach the hair from the fruits, discard the fruits, and dry the hair.

Properties　　Root: slightly bitter and astringent tasting; cool. Anti-inflammatory. Fruit hair: Bland tasting; neutral, toxic. Vermifuge, purgative.

Indications　　Root: 1. Acute and chronic dysentery; 2. Sore throat. Use 10 gm. as decoction. Fruit hair; Vermifuge for ascaris, pinworm, strongyloides. Also as purgative. Use 3-5 gm., grind into fine powder and take internally. Leaves: use externally in boils, ulcers, and wound bleeding.

Prescription　　Indolent ulcers: Mallotus philipinensis leaves boiled in water for washing, and also grind leaves into powder for applying to lesion.

Remarks　　The fruits and the red powdery spots under the leaves are poisonous. Main signs of poisoning are nausea, vomiting, and severe diarrhea.

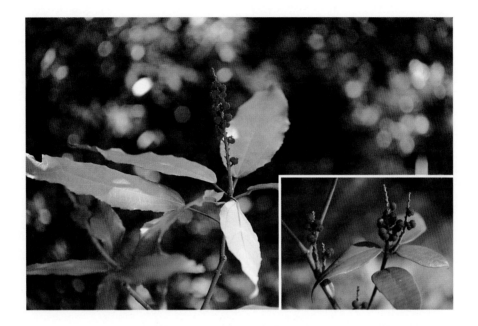

　　大戟科、野桐屬之常綠小喬木，高約10米。嫩莖被褐色星狀柔毛。葉互生，卵形、寬卵形至披針形；基出脈3條；葉背密被短星狀毛及紅色腺點；葉基有2腺體；葉柄密被短柔毛。雌雄同株異花；花小，無花瓣；總狀花序頂生或腋生，常有分枝，花序枝及花梗密被星狀毛及腺點。雄花萼片外被星狀茸毛及腺點，雄蕊多數；子房被鮮紅色腺點。蒴果密被紅色腺點及星狀毛。花期：四月至五月。

Euphorbiaceae: Evergreen small trees, up to 10m high. Branchlets brown stellate pubescent. Leaves alternate, ovate, broad ovate or lanceolate; trinervious; covered densely with stellate hairs and red glands beneath; base with two glands; petiole densely pubescent. Flowers minute, petals none, unisexual, monoecious, racemes axillary or terminal, often branching; infloresence and pedicels densely covered with stellate hairs and granular glands; male flower sepals covered with stellate hairs and granular glands on the outside, stamens numerous; ovaries covered with scarlet glands. Capsules densely covered with red glands and stellate tomentum. Flowering from April to May.

白 粉 藤

Cissus repens Lam.

別　　名　接骨藤、粉藤薯、獨腳烏桕。

生長環境　生於山坡、溝谷灌木叢中。

採集加工　藥用根、莖、葉。全年可採，曬乾或鮮用。

性味功能　根：味淡、微辛，性涼。清熱，消腫。莖、葉：味苦，性寒。有小毒。拔毒消腫。

主治用法　根：1. 頸淋巴結結核；2. 風濕骨痛；3. 腎炎。每用 3 至 5 錢，水煎服。莖、葉：多外用於瘡瘍腫毒，蛇咬傷。鮮品適量，搗敷或煎水洗患處。

方　　例　風濕骨痛：白粉藤、金櫻子、五指毛桃，均用根各1兩，煲豬尾，飲湯食肉。

Habitat　　　On slopes, ravines, and in thickets.

Preparation　　Use roots, stems, leaves. Collect all year round, dry under sun or use fresh.

Properties　　Roots: bland and acrid tasting; cool. Anti-inflammatory; reduce swelling. Stem, leaves: Bitter tasting; cold, slightly toxic. Drain toxins and reduce swelling.

Indications　　Roots: 1. Tuberculous lymphadenopathy of the neck; 2. Rheumatic bone pain; 3. Nephritis. Use 10-15 gm., as decoction. Stem and leaves: Mostly used externally for furunculosis, snake bites. Use fresh herb as poultice or boil in water for washing.

Prescriptions　Rheumatic bone pain: Cissus repens, Rosa laevigata, Ficus hirta, all using root, 30 gm. each, cook with pork tail, consume soup and meat.

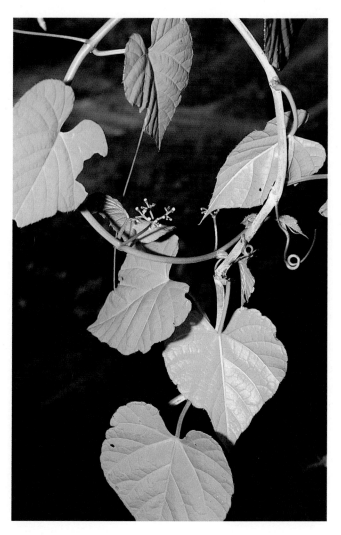

　　葡萄科、白粉藤屬之草質藤本，有捲鬚以利攀援。莖上有白粉，樹皮之皮孔明顯，嫩莖帶微紅色，莖橫切面可見白色之髓部。葉互生，葉片心狀卵形或狹卵形；葉緣有微紅色小齒 10 餘個。聚傘花序，花小，輻射對稱；花萼小；花瓣 4 片，分生，鑷合狀排列；雄蕊 4 枚，與花瓣對生，着生於花盤基部；花盤明顯；子房上位；柱頭小。漿果。種子具豐富胚乳，胚細小。花期：七月。

Vitaceae: Herbal vines with tendrils for climbing. Stem covered with white powder, lenticels prominent, young branches slightly reddish, white medulla visible in the transverse section of stem. Leaves alternate, cordate-ovate or narrow ovate; margins with ten-odd slightly reddish small teeth. Flowers small, radially symmetrical, cymose; sepals small; petals 4, distinct, valvate; stamens 4, opposite to petals, arising from the base of the prominent disc; ovary superior; stigmas minute. Berry. Seeds with thick endosperm, embryo small. Flowering in July.

三 葉 青

Tetrastigma hemsleyanum Diels et Gilg

別　　名　蛇附子、金綫吊葫蘆、石老鼠、石猴子、三葉扁藤、三葉崖爬藤。

生長環境　生於山谷疏林中或石壁上陰處。

採集加工　藥用塊根或全草。全年可採，曬乾或鮮用。

性味功能　味微苦，性平。清熱解毒，活血止痛。

主治用法　1. 小兒高熱驚厥；2. 病毒性腦膜炎；3. 扁桃體炎，白喉；4. 肝炎，腎炎；5. 風濕關節痛，坐骨神經痛。每用3至5錢，水煎服。外用治毒蛇咬傷，淋巴結結核，子宮頸炎，癰瘡腫毒，跌打損傷。鮮品適量，酒或水磨糊搽患處。

方　　例　1. 小兒高熱：三葉青塊根1錢，鈎藤、重樓根各2錢，水煎服。

2. 病毒性腦膜炎：三葉青塊根5錢（小童3錢），水煎服。

3. 急、慢性腎炎：三葉青鮮根1兩，與青殼鴨蛋同煮熟服。

主要成分　含氨基酸、有機酸、酚類、地衣糖、油脂（萜類）。

附　　註　本品具有很強的促進白血球吞噬細菌作用。

Habitat　　In ravines, woods, or shady areas of rocky walls.

Preparation　　Use tuber or whole herb. Collect all year round, dry under sun or use fresh.

Properties　　Slightly bitter tasting; neutral. Anti-inflammatory, analgesic; promotes circulation.

Indications　　1. Infantile febrile convulsion; 2. Viral encephalitis; 3. Tonsillitis, diphtheria; 4. Hepatitis, nephritis; 5. Rheumatic arthritis, sciatica. Use 10-15 gm., as decoction. External use in snake bites, tuberculous lymphadenopathy, cervicitis, furuncles and carbuncles, traumatic injury. Grind fresh herb with added wine for topical application.

Prescriptions　　1. High fever in infants: Tetrastigma hemsleyanum tuber 3 gm., Uncaria hirsuta, Paris chinensis, 6 gm. each, as decoction.

2. Viral encephalitis: Tetrastigma hemsleyanum 15 gm. (10 gm. for children), as decoction.

Remarks　　This herb promotes phagocytosis of the white blood cells intensely.

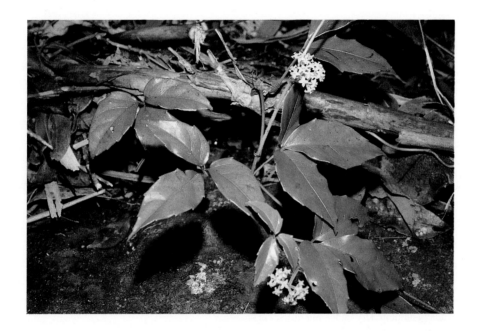

　　葡萄科、崖爬藤屬之攀援藤本，莖細弱。捲鬚不分枝。掌狀複葉，小葉3片，草質；中間小葉稍大，卵狀披針形，葉前端短漸尖或漸尖，葉緣疏生小鋸齒；側生2小葉之葉基偏斜。聚傘花序腋生，花序梗比葉柄短；花小，黃綠色；花梗有短硬毛；花盤明顯，有齒；花瓣4，近卵形，頂端有不明顯之小角；柱頭無柄，裂片4，星狀開裂。漿果球形，紅褐色，成熟時黑色。花期：四月至五月。

Vitaceae: Climbing lianas, stems delicate. Tendrils undivided. Leaves herbaceous; trifoliolate, the middle leaflet larger, ovate-lanceolate, apex short-acuminate or acuminate, sparsely serrulate; the lateral leaflets with oblique base. Flowers small, yellowish-green, in axillary cymes, rachis of the inflorescence shorter than petiole; pedicels short hispid; discs prominent, toothed; petals 4, subovate, tip with inconspicuous protuberances; stigma sessile, 4-lobed, star-shaped. Berries globose, reddish-brown, black at maturity. Flowering from April to May.

南 蛇 藤

Celastrus orbiculatus Thunb.

別　　名　地南蛇、過山楓、南蛇風、黃果藤。

生長環境　生於山坡灌木叢中。

採集加工　藥用全株。根、藤全年可採，葉夏季採，果秋季採，曬乾或鮮用。

性味功能　根、藤：味辛，性溫；祛風濕，活血。果：味甘、苦，性平；安神鎮靜。葉：味苦，性平。全株均有小毒。解毒散瘀。

主治用法　根、藤：風濕性關節炎，腰腿痛，跌打損傷。果：神經衰弱，心悸，失眠。葉：跌打損傷，多發性癤腫，蛇咬傷。每用根、藤3至5錢，果2至5錢，水煎服。孕婦忌服。葉外用適量，搗敷患處。

方　　例　風濕筋骨痛，關節痛，腰痛：南蛇藤、凌霄花各4兩，八角楓根2兩。白酒半斤，浸七天。每日睡前服5錢。

主要成分　葉含山奈甙（kaempferitrin）。根皮含一種具抗吉田肉瘤活性的紅色結晶。種子含脂肪油47.07-58.69%。

Habitat　　In thickets on slopes.

Preparation　　Use whole herb. Collect roots and vines all year round, leaves in summer, fruits in autumn. Dry under sun or use fresh.

Properties　　Roots, vines: Acrid tasting; warm. Anti-rheumatic, promote circulation. Fruits: Sweet and bitter tasting; neutral. Sedative. Leaves: Bitter tasting; neutral. Anti-inflammatory; resolve ecchymosis. The whole herb is slightly toxic.

Indications　　Roots, vines: rheumatic arthritis, knee and back pain, traumatic injury. Fruits: Neurasthenia, palpitation, insomnia. Leaves: traumatic injury, furunculosis, snake bites. Use roots, vines, 10-15 gm., fruits 5-15 gm., as decoction. Contraindicated in pregnancy. Mash leaves for external use.

Prescription　　Rheumatic arthralgia, bone pains, low back pains: Celastrus orbiculatus, Campsis grandiflora flowers, each 120 gm., Alangium chinense roots 60 gm., immerse in half catty (300 gm.) of white wine for seven days. Take 15 gm. of this at bedtimes.

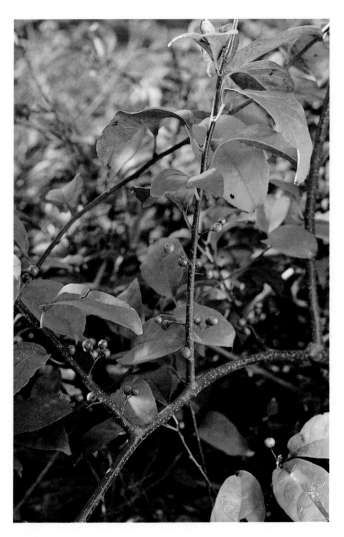

　　衛矛科、南蛇藤屬之藤狀灌
木；嫩莖上有多數皮孔。葉互生，
寬橢圓。倒卵形或近圓形；葉頂端
有小尖頭，葉基寬楔形。聚傘花序
頂生及腋生，有花 5 至 7 朵，花梗
短；花雜性，黃綠色；雄花 5 數，
雄蕊着生於杯狀花盤之邊緣，退化
雌蕊柱狀；雌花之雄蕊不育，子房
基部被杯狀花盤所包圍，花柱細
長，柱頭 3 裂，而裂端再 2 淺裂。蒴
果黃色，3 裂。種子具紅色之肉質
假種皮。花期：四月。

Celastraceae: Twining shrubs;
stems with numerous lenticels when
young. Leaves alternate, broad elliptic,
obovate or suborbicular; apex
mucronate, base cuneiform. Flowers
polygamous, yellowish-green, pedicels
short, 5-7 flowered in terminal or axillary
cymes; male flowers 5-merous, stamens
at the margin of cupular floral-disc,
pistillodes columnar; stamens sterile in
female flowers, stigma 3-lobed, with
each lobe again shallowly 2-lobed.
Capsules yellow, 3 lobed. Aril fleshy,
red. Flowering in April.

疏 花 衛 矛

Euonymus laxiflorus Champ.

別　　名　土杜仲、木杜仲、山杜仲、大丁黃、五稔子、絲棉木。

生長環境　生於灌木叢中。

採集加工　藥用根、樹皮和葉。全年可採，曬乾用。

性味功能　味淡、澀，性平。祛風濕，強筋骨。

主治用法　1. 腰骨酸痛；2. 跌打，骨折；3. 慢性腎炎。每用 5 錢至 1 兩，水煎或泡酒服。外用葉適量，研末調敷，治骨折，跌打外傷。

方　　例　1. 腰膝酸痛：疏花衛矛根 1 兩，加豬尾骨適量，同燉服。

2. 慢性腎炎：疏花衛矛根、土牛膝、車前草各 5 錢，加瘦肉適量同燉，服湯食肉。

附　　註　同屬植物華衛矛（Euonymus chinensis）功效與本種近似。

Habitat　　In thickets.

Preparation　　Use roots, bark, and leaves. Collect all year round, dry under sun.

Properties　　Bland and astringent tasting, neutral. Anti-rheumatic. Strengthens muscles and joints.

Indications　　1. Low back aches; 2. Traumatic injury, fractures; 3. Chronic nephritis. Use 15-30 gm., as decoction or soak in wine. For external use, grind into powder and use as poultice in fractures and traumatic injury.

Prescriptions　　1. Loin and leg pains: Euonymus laxiflorus roots 30 gm., boiled with pork tail bones as soup.

2. Chronic nephritis: Euonymus laxiflorus, Achyranthes aspera, Plantago major, 15 gm. each, cook with pork to make soup.

Remarks　　Another plant of the same genus, Euonymus chinensis, has similar medicinal effects.

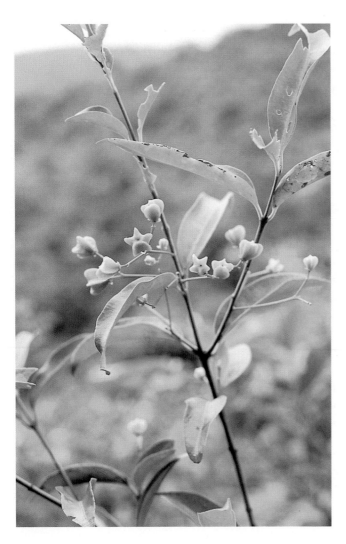

衛矛科、衛矛屬之常綠灌木，高可達5米。葉對生，薄革質，卵形、橢圓形至狹橢圓形；葉頂端漸尖至長漸尖，葉基截形；葉緣有淺鋸齒或近全緣；側脈不明顯，且少而疏。聚傘花序有花5至9朵；花紫紅色至淡紅色，直徑約1厘米，5數，雄蕊無花絲，雌蕊無花柱。蒴果紫紅色，倒錐形，先端平截，有5淺裂。種子紅褐色；假種皮紅色，杯狀，只包圍種子基部約1/4。花期：五月。

Celastraceae: Evergreen shrubs, up to 5m high. Leaves opposite, thin coriaceous, ovate, elliptic or narrow elliptic; apex acuminate or long-acuminate, base cuneiform; margin serrulate or nearly entire; lateral veins inconspicuous and sparse. Flowers carmine to reddish, about 1cm in diameter, 5-merous, 5-9 flowered in cymes; stamens without filaments, pistils without styles. Capsules carmine, truncated obconic, shallowly 5-lobed. Seeds reddish-brown; aril red, cupular, covering only one quarter of the seed. Flowering in May.

黃　槿

Hibiscus tiliaceus L.

別　　名　右納、海麻、海羅樹、鹽水面頭果。

生長環境　生於海邊，或栽培為防潮、防風樹。

採集加工　藥用葉、樹皮、花。四季可採，多作鮮用。

性味功能　味甘、淡，性微寒。清熱解毒，止咳。

主治用法　1. 支氣管炎咳嗽；2. 發熱；3. 木薯中毒。每用 1 至 2 兩，水煎服。外用治瘡癧腫毒；鮮嫩葉或樹皮適量，搗爛外敷患處。

方　　例　1. 支氣管炎咳嗽：黃槿鮮嫩葉 1 至 2 兩，水煎加糖服。

2. 木薯中毒：鮮花或嫩葉 1 至 2 兩，搗爛取汁沖白糖水服，重者可日服 2 至 3 劑。

附　　註　黃槿嫩枝葉可供蔬食，根有催吐作用。

Habitat　　Along seaside, or planted to break tides and wind.

Preparation　　Use bark, leaves, and flowers. Collect all year round, use fresh.

Properties　　Sweet and bland tasting; slightly cold. Anti-inflammatory, antitussive.

Indications　　1. Bronchitis and cough; 2. Fever; 3. Cassava poisoning. Use 30-60 gm., as decoction. External use in boils and abscesses, by applying mashed fresh leaves or bark to affected parts.

Prescriptions　　1. Bronchitic coughs: Hibiscus tiliaceus leaves 30-60 gm., brew in water and take with some sugar.

2. Cassava poisoning: Fresh flowers or tender leaves 30-60 gm., mash to get the sap, dilute, and take with sugar. In severe cases, doses can be repeated 2-3 times daily.

Remarks　　The tender leaves and stem can be eaten as vegetable. The root has emetic action.

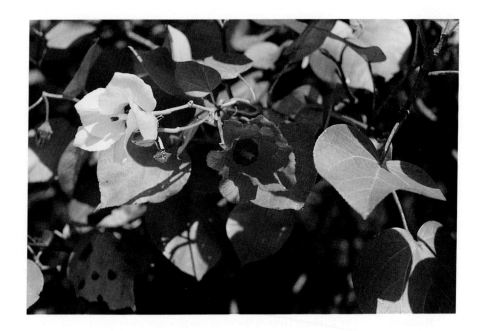

　　錦葵科、木槿屬之常綠灌木或小喬木，高約10米。樹皮灰白色。葉互生，革質，近圓形；葉頂端急尖，葉基心形；葉背灰白色，且密生星狀絨毛；托葉早落。花頂生或腋生，常由數花組成聚傘花序；小苞片7至10，條狀披針形，中部以下連合成杯狀；萼片5，披針形，基部1/4處合生；花冠黃色，直徑約7厘米，花美麗。蒴果卵圓形，5瓣裂，果瓣木質。種子多數，表面平滑。花期：六月至七月。

　　Malvaceae: Evergreen shrubs or small trees, up to 10m high. Barks pale gray. Leaves alternate, coriaceous, suborbicular; apex acute, base cordate; pale and densely pubescent with stellate hairs beneath; stipules shed off early. Flowers beautiful, several flowers in terminal or axillary cymes; bracteoles 7-10, linear-lanceolate, lower part united to form a cup; sepals 5, lanceolate, base 1/4 connate; corolla yellow, diameter about 7cm. Capsule ovoid, 5-valved dehiscent, valves woody. Seeds numerous, surface smooth. Flowering from June to July.

刺 果 藤

Byttneria aspera Colebr.

別　　名　　大膠藤、牛蹄麻、雞冠麻。

生長環境　　生於山谷林中或溪邊。

採集加工　　藥用根或莖。全年可採，切段，曬乾或鮮用。

性味功能　　味澀、微苦，性微溫。祛風濕，壯筋骨。

主治用法　　1. 產後筋骨痛；2. 風濕骨痛，腰肌勞損。每用根 5 錢至 1 兩，水煎服。外用治跌打骨折，鮮根適量搗爛，酒炒外敷患處。

附　　註　　本品莖皮纖維可製繩索。

Habitat　　In valleys, woods, or by creek sides.

Preparation　　Use roots or stems. Collect all year round, cut into segments, dry under sun or use fresh.

Properties　　Astringent and slightly bitter tasting; mildly warm. Anti-rheumatic; strengthens muscles and joints.

Indications　　1. Postpartum aches and pains; 2. Rheumatic bone pains, low back pains. Use roots 15-30 gm., as decoction. External use in traumatic injury or fractures, mash fresh roots and fry with wine for topical poultice.

Remarks　　The stem covering of the vines can be made into ropes.

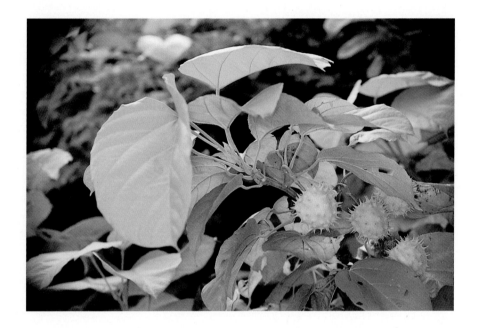

　　梧桐科、刺果藤屬之木質藤本。小枝上密生緊貼的微柔毛。葉寬卵至卵形，長及寬略等長，葉先端短漸尖或微鈍，葉基心形，葉背密被白色星狀短柔毛。圓錐花序長達10厘米，花朵在花序分枝上呈傘形排列；萼片5，三角形，密被微柔毛；花瓣5片，較萼片長，外面白色，內面粉紅色；雄蕊合生成筒狀。蒴果圓球形，直徑3至4厘米，具多數短粗刺及短柔毛。花期：八月。

　　Sterculiaceae: Woody lianas. Branches densely pilose. Leaves broad-ovate to ovate, length and width about equal, apex short-acuminate or slightly obtuse, base cordate, densely covered with short, fine, white stellate hairs beneath. Panicles up to 10cm long, with each peduncle bearing umbellate flowers; sepals 5, deltoid, densely pilose; petals 5, longer than sepals, white outside, pink inside; stamens connate, tubular. Capsules globose, 3-4cm in diameter, covered with numerous short, thick prickles and short fine hairs. Flowering in August.

假 蘋 婆

Sterculia lanceolata Cav.

別　　名　賽蘋婆、雞冠木、紅郎傘、假苹婆。

生長環境　生於山谷、水澗邊。

採集加工　藥用樹皮、葉。全年可採，曬乾或鮮用。

性味功能　味辛，性溫。散瘀，止痛。

主治用法　葉：跌打損傷，瘀血疼痛。樹皮：白帶，淋濁。每用3至5錢，水煎
服。外用適量。

附　　註　莖皮纖維可作麻袋的原料，也可造紙。

Habitat　　　In ravines, along streams.

Preparation　Use bark and leaves. Collect all year round, dry under sun or use fresh.

Properties　Acrid tasting; warm. Resorbs bruises; analgesic.

Indications　Leaves: traumatic injury, painful bruises. Bark: leucorrhea. Use 10-15 gm., as decoction. For external application, use suitable amounts.

Remarks　　Fibres from the stems can be used to make sacks.

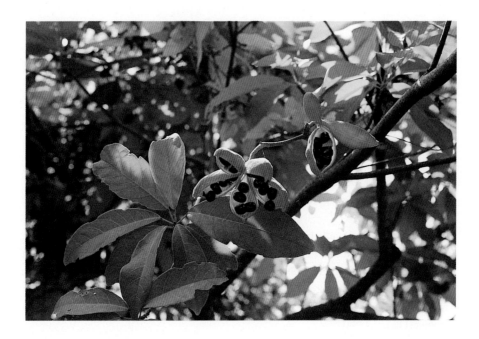

　　梧桐科、蘋婆屬之常綠喬木，高約7米。小枝常彎曲。樹冠之葉甚密。葉近革質，橢圓狀矩圓形，長可達20厘米。圓錐花序腋生；花細小不顯眼，綠或粉紅色，雜性，無花冠；萼粉紅色；花藥10枚生於雄蕊柱頂端呈球形；子房密生短柔毛。蓇葖2至5，組成星形之果，密生微柔毛，幼時綠色，繼而變黃、橙紅，成熟時成顯眼之鮮紅色，並於下緣開裂露出黑色種子。花期：四月至五月。

　　Sterculiaceae: Evergreen trees, up to 7m high. Branches often bending. Crown dense. Leaves subcoriaceous, elliptic-oblong, up to 20cm long. flowers minute, inconspicuous, green or pink, corolla non-existent, polygamous in axillary panicles; sepals pink; anthers 10, forming a globule at the tip of the stamen; ovary densely pilose. Follicles 2-5, forming star-shaped fruits, densely pilose, green when young, becoming yellow, orange, then conspicuously scarlet at maturity. Seeds exposed as the pods break open at the lower margins. Flowering from April to May.

水 東 哥

Saurauia tristyla DC.

別　　名　水枇杷、山枇杷、紅毛樹、米花樹、白凡木。

生長環境　生於山谷、溪邊或林下陰濕處。

採集加工　藥用根、樹皮和葉。秋、冬季採收，切片，曬乾。

性味功能　味微苦，性涼。清熱解毒，止咳，止痛。

主治用法　根：風熱咳嗽，風火牙痛，白帶，尿路感染，精神分裂症，肝炎。樹皮：尿路感染，外用於骨髓炎，癰癤。葉外用於燒燙傷。每用 3 至 5 錢，水煎服。

方　　例　燒燙傷：葉研粉，麻油調敷患處。

Habitat　　In ravines, by creek sides, or under woods in damp shady soil.

Preparation　Use roots, bark, and leaves. Collect in autumn and winter, slice, dry under sun.

Properties　Slightly bitter tasting; cool. Anti-inflammatory, antitussive, analgesic.

Indications　Roots: Fever and coughs, toothache, leucorrhea, urinary tract infection, schizophrenia, hepatitis. Bark: Urinary tract infection, external use in osteomyelitis, carbunculosis. Leaves useful in burns and scalds. Use 10-15 gm., as decoction.

Prescription　Burns and scalds: Grind leaves into fine powder and blend with sesame oil for topical use.

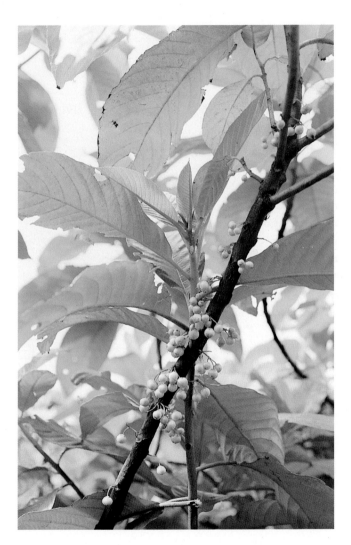

獼猴桃科、水東哥屬之灌木或小喬木。嫩莖有鏽色鱗片狀伏毛，長大則毛漸脫落。葉互生，矩圓形、倒卵狀矩圓形或寬橢圓形；幼時有稀疏鱗片狀糙伏毛，後變無毛；葉長可達28厘米。聚傘花序腋生或生於老莖之葉痕腋部，有總花梗；花淡紅色；萼片5片，卵形；花瓣5片，基部合生，上部向外反折；雄蕊多數；子房卵形，花柱上部有數分枝。漿果近球形。種子多數，細小。花期：五月。

Actinidiaceae: Shrubs or small trees. Young stems with rust- and scale-like pubescences which fall off on aging. Leaves alternate, oblong, obovate-oblong or broad elliptic; sparsely scaly-strigose when young, later becoming glabrous, up to 28cm long. Flowers reddish, in axillary cymes with peduncles; sepals 5, ovate; petals 5, connate at base, upper part reflexed; stamens numerous; ovary ovoid, tip of styles split. Berry subglobose. Seeds numerous, small. Flowering in May.

黃　瑞　木

Adinandra millettii (Hook. et Arn.) Benth.

別　　名　　毛藥紅淡、烏珠子、楊桐、雞仔茶。

生長環境　　生於山坡、路旁灌木叢中。

採集加工　　藥用根、嫩葉。根全年可採，嫩葉夏、秋採，曬乾或鮮用。

性味功能　　味甘、微苦，性涼。解毒，止血。

主治用法　　1. 肝炎，腮腺炎；2. 鼻衄，尿血。每用根1至2兩，水煎服。外用治瘡癤，蛇咬傷，毒蜂螫傷，鮮嫩葉適量，搗爛外敷。

方　　例　　1. 慢性肝炎：黃瑞木根、黑豆各2兩，水煎服。

2. 鼻衄（鼻出血）：黃瑞木根、梔子根各2兩，水煎服。

Habitat　　On slopes and in roadside thickets.

Preparation　　Use roots and young leaves. Collect roots all year round, young leaves in summer and autumn, dry under sun or use fresh.

Properties　　Sweet, slightly bitter tasting; cool. Anti-inflammatory, haemostatic.

Indications　　1. Hepatitis, parotitis; 2. Epistaxis, hematuria. Use roots 30-60 gm., as decoction. Extenal use in boils, snake bites, bee stings. Mash fresh leaves for local use.

Prescriptions　　1. Chronic hepatitis: Adinandra millettii roots, and black beans, 60 gm. each, as decoction.

2. Epistaxia: Adinandra millettii roots, Gardenia jasminoides roots, 60 gm. each, as decoction.

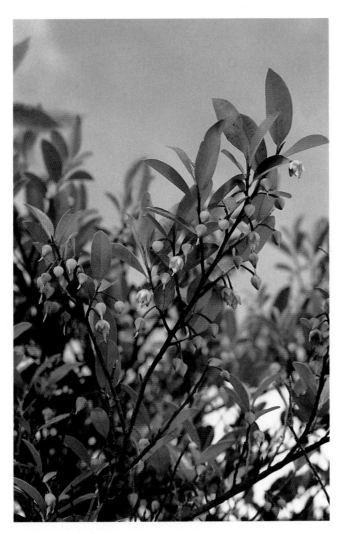

山茶科、紅淡屬之灌木或小喬木。幼莖及頂芽疏生柔毛。葉互生，革質，矩圓狀橢圓形，全緣；幼葉有密集的柔毛，長大後無毛。花單獨腋生，白色，花梗幼細；萼片 5，卵狀三角形，具細腺齒和睫毛；花冠裂片 5；雄蕊約 25，花藥密生白色柔毛；子房 3 室，具白色柔毛；花柱無毛。果近球形，漿果，直徑7至8毫米，有柔毛或近無毛。種子細小，黑色有亮澤。花期：四月至五月。

Theaceae: Shrubs or small trees. Young branches and terminal buds sparsely pilose. Leaves alternate, Leathery, oblong-elliptic, margins entire; young leaves densely pilose, glabrous at maturity. Flowers white, solitary, axillary, pedicel slender; sepals 5, ovate-deltoid, possessing fine glandular teeth and ciliate hairs; corolla segments 5; stamens about 25, anthers densely white pilose, ovary 3-chambered, white pilose; styles glabrous. Fruits berries, subglobose, diameter 7-8 mm, pilose or near glabrous. Seeds minute, black, shiny. Flowering from April to May.

米 碎 花

Eurya chinensis R. Brown

別　　名　崗茶、梅養東、蝦辣眼。

生長環境　生於山坡草地、灌木叢中。

採集加工　藥用全株或根。全年可採，曬乾或鮮用。

性味功能　味甘、淡、微澀，性涼。清熱解毒。

主治用法　預防流行性感冒，每用5錢至1兩，水煎服。外用治燒、燙傷，膿疱瘡，適量煎水洗，或研粉，麻油調敷患處。

方　　例　膿疱瘡：米碎花、金銀花各5錢，水煎服，和外洗患處。

Habitat　　　　On grassland along slopes and in thickets.

Preparation　　Use whole herb or roots. Collect all year round, dry under sun or use fresh.

Properties　　Sweet and bland, slightly astringent tasting; cool. Anti-inflammatory.

Indications　　Prevention of epidemic influenza. Use 15-30 gm., as decoction. External use in burns and scalds, impetigo. Boil suitable amount in water for washing, or pulverize and blend with sesame oil for topical use.

Remarks　　　Impetigo: Eurya chinensis, Lonicera japonica, 15 gm. each, as decoction and also for washing the lesion.

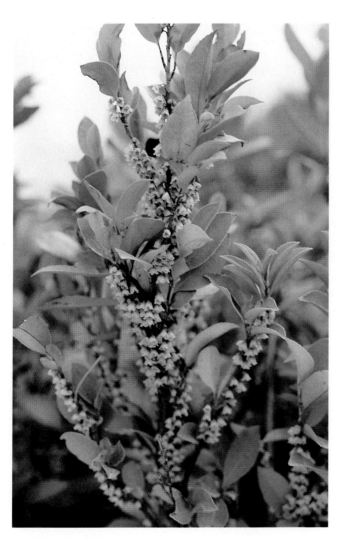

　　山茶科、柃木屬之小灌木。嫩莖有棱，頂芽及嫩莖均被短柔毛。葉互生，薄革質，倒卵形至倒卵狀橢圓形，葉緣密生細鋸齒。雌雄異株，花細小，白色至黃綠色，1至4朵叢生；萼片卵形；雄花苞片細小，花瓣倒卵形，雄蕊約15，1輪；雌花花瓣卵形，子房無毛，花柱頂端3淺裂。果實圓球形，直徑約4毫米，熟時黑色；種子細小，有網狀紋凸起。花期：十二月。

Theaceae: Small shrubs. Young stems ridged, terminal buds and young stems pilose. Leaves alternate, thin coriaceous, obovate or obovate-elliptic, serrulate. Dioecious, flowers small, white or yellowish-green, 1-4 clustered; sepals ovate; staminate bracts small, petals obovate, stamens about 15 in one whorl; pistillate petals ovate, ovary hairless, styles shallowly trifid. Fruits globose, 4mm in diameter, black at maturity; seeds minute, with reticulate ridges on the surface. Flowering in December.

木　荷

Schima superba Gardn. et Champ.

別　　名　木艾樹、何樹、柯樹、回樹。

生長環境　生於向陽山地樹林中。

採集加工　藥用根皮及葉。全年可採，曬乾用。

性味功能　味苦，性溫。有大毒。清熱解毒。

主治用法　根皮：外敷疔瘡，無名腫毒。葉：爛腿，瘡毒。本品有大毒，只供外敷，不可內服。

附　　註　據報導，伐木者常因皮膚與樹皮(內皮)接觸引起紅腫、發癢。可用清水、茶葉水或硼酸溶液洗滌。

Habitat　　　In woods on sunny slopes.

Preparation　Use root skins and leaves. Collect all year round, dry under sun.

Properties　Bitter tasting; warm. Very toxic, anti-inflammatory.

Indications　Root skins: External use in furuncles, and pyoderma. Leaves: Leg sores, boils. This herb is very toxic and should only be used externally.

Remarks　　Contact dermatitis from this tree is frequently suffered by woodcutters, resulting in erythema, swelling, and pruritus. This can be alleviated by washing with water, tea, or boric acid solution.

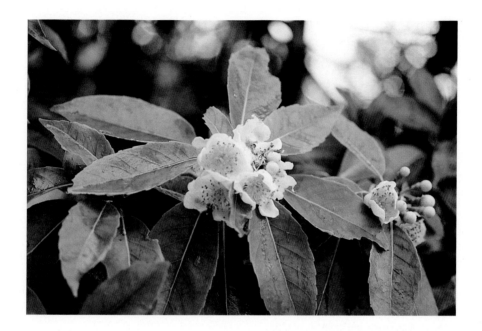

　　山茶科、木荷屬之喬木，高可達18米。樹莖質堅硬，嫩莖無毛或於頂端附近有細毛。
葉互生，革質，卵狀橢圓形至矩圓形，葉緣近無齒；葉前端漸尖，葉基楔形。花白色，單獨
腋生或頂生成總狀花序；花梗通常直立；萼片5片，邊緣有細毛；花瓣5片，倒卵形；雄蕊
多數，花藥T字形着生於雄蕊頂；子房基部密生細毛。蒴果扁球形，直徑約 1.5 厘米，5
裂。種子周圍有翅。花期：四月至五月。

　　Theaceae: Trees, up to 18m high, trunk hard, young stems glabrous or with fine hairs near the
tips. Leaves alternate, coriaceous, ovate-elliptic to oblong, margin sub-entire; apex acuminate, base
cuneate. Flowers white, solitary axillary or in racemes terminally; pedicels usually erect; sepals 5,
margin hairy, petals 5, obovate; stamens numerous, anthers versatile; ovary densely pilose at base.
Capsules compressed globose, about 1.5cm in diameter, 5-valved. Seeds winged. Flowering from April
to May.

菫　菜

Viola arcuata Bl.

別　　名　白犁頭草。

生長環境　生於路旁、山邊草坡上。

採集加工　藥用全草。春、夏採收，曬乾或鮮用。

性味功能　味辛、酸，性寒。清熱解毒。

主治用法　1. 瘡癤，急性乳腺炎；2. 急性結膜炎；3. 跌打腫痛。每用3至5錢，水煎服。外用鮮品適量，搗爛敷患處。

方　　例　瘡癤，急性乳腺炎：菫菜、蒲公英、金銀花各5錢，水煎服。外用鮮菫菜適量加紅糖少許，搗爛敷患處。

Habitat　　On roadside, hillside lawns.

Preparation　　Use whole herb. Collect in spring and summer. Dry under sun or use fresh.

Properties　　Acrid and sour tasting; cold. Anti-inflammatory.

Indications　　1. Furuncles, acute mastitis; 2. Acute conjunctivitis; 3. Traumatic injury. Use 10-15 gm., as decoction. For external use, mash fresh herb as poultice.

Prescription　　Boils, acute mastitis: Viola arcuata, Taraxacum mongolicum, Lonicera japonica flower buds, 15 gm. each, as decoction. For external use, mix fresh Viola arcuata with brown sugar, mash and apply as poultice.

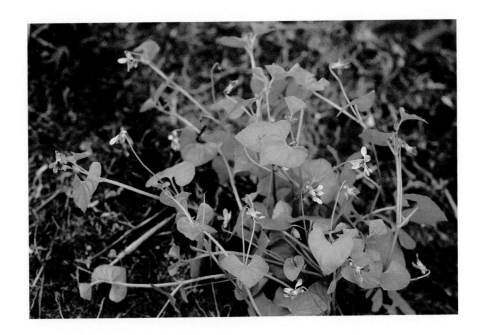

　　菫菜科、菫菜屬之直立草本，高約15厘米，地下莖很短。根宿存，長圓錐形。葉分基
生葉及莖生葉兩種：前者較多，具淡綠色微帶紅之長葉柄；後者較少，疏生於纖弱之莖上，
具披針形或條狀披針形之托葉；兩者之葉片皆闊心形或近圓形，葉片深綠色，葉緣具淺圓鈍
齒。花細小，粉紅色帶黃，基生或腋生；萼片及花瓣5數；距短。蒴果。花期：九月。

Violaceae: Herbs, erect, 15cm high, underground stems very short. Roots persistent, elongated conic. Leaves two types: basal or cauline, the former being more numerous, with long, pale greenish-red petioles, and the latter less, sparsely scattered on delicate stems, with lanceolate or linear-lanceolate stipules; laminae for both types of leaves broadly cordate or subcordate, dark greenish, margins crenulate. Flowers small, pink with patches of yellow, basal or axillary; sepals and petals 5-merous; spurs short. Capsules. Flowering in September.

紅 千 層

Callistemon rigidus R. Br.

生長環境　多為栽培。

採集加工　藥用葉。全年可採，陰乾。

性味功能　味辛，性微溫。解表祛風。

主治用法　1.感冒；2.風濕痛。每用3至5錢，水煎服。外用治濕疹，跌打損傷。鮮品適量，搗敷，或煎水洗患處。

主要成分　葉含揮發油。

Habitat　　Mostly cultivated.

Preparation　　Use leaves. Collect all year round. Dry under shade.

Properties　　Acrid tasting, slightly warm. Effective against colds.

Indications　　1. Common cold; 2. Rheumatic pain. Use 10-15 gm., as decoction. External use in eczema, traumatic injury. Mash fresh herb as poultice, or boil in water for washing.

Remarks　　Leaves contain aromatic oils.

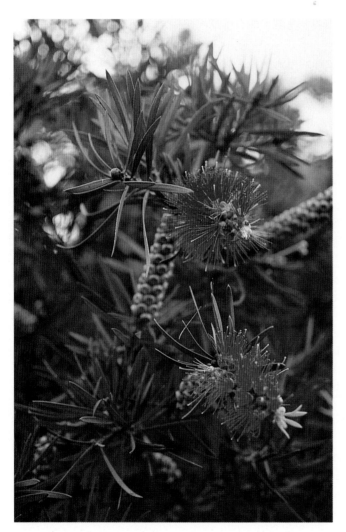

　　姚金娘科、紅千層屬之常綠小喬木。樹皮暗灰色，幼枝及嫩葉被白色柔毛。葉互生，條形，堅硬而尖，有透明腺點，中脈明顯，無葉柄。穗狀花序稠密，生近枝頂，花序軸向上繼續生成一有葉之正常莖；花紅色；萼管被毛，基部與子房貼生，裂片5；花瓣5，圓形，有透明腺點；雄蕊多數，鮮紅色，比花瓣長；雌蕊花柱長，綠色，頂端鮮紅色。蒴果半球形，頂端截平。花期：五月。

Myrtaceae: Evergreen trees. Bark dull grey, twigs and young leaves white pilose. Leaves alternate, linear, firm and cuspidate, with transparent glands, sessile, mid-rib conspicuous. Flowers red, borne densely in subterminal spikes, upper part of rachis continuing its growth to become a normal shoot with leaves; sepals 5, tubular, hairy, base connate with ovary; petals 5, orbicular, with transparent glands; stamens numerous, bright red, longer than petals, styles long, green, bright red at tip. Capsules hemispheric, tip truncated. Flowering in May.

石榴（安石榴）

Punica granatum L.

別　　名　石榴殼、若榴、丹若、金罌、酸石榴皮、榭榴。

生長環境　多栽培於庭園。

採集加工　藥用果皮為主，全株均可入藥。果實夏、秋採，取果皮曬乾用。

性味功能　味酸、澀，性溫。收斂止瀉，止血，驅蟲。

主治用法　1. 慢性腹瀉，痢疾；2. 便血，脫肛；3. 崩漏，白帶；4. 蟲積腹痛。每用果皮 3 至 5 錢，水煎服。外用治稻田性皮炎，燙傷。煎水浸洗或研末外敷。

方　　例　1. 慢性腹瀉：石榴皮 5 錢，肉豆蔻（去油）3 錢，水煎服。

2. 慢性痢疾：石榴皮、白頭翁、馬齒莧、車前草各 5 錢，水煎服。

3. 縧蟲、蛔蟲：石榴皮、檳榔研細末，每次服 2 錢，每日兩次，連服二天。

主要成分　果皮含大量鞣質，並含黏液質等。根及莖皮含生物鹼 0.3-0.5%。

附　　註　石榴根、莖皮有毒，作用似石榴皮，宜慎用；葉用於急性腸炎；花用於吐血，衄血；果實煎汁可作扁桃腺炎，咽喉炎，口腔炎的含漱劑。

Habitat　　Mostly cultivated in gardens (as pomegranate).

Preparation　　Use the rind of fruits or the whole herb. Collect fruits in summer and autumn, remove rind to dry under sun.

Properties　　Sour and astringent tasting; warm. Anti-diarrheal, heamostatic, vermifuge.

Indications　　1. Chronic diarrhea, dysentery; 2. Rectal bleeding, rectal prolapse. 3. Massive uterine bleeding, leucorrhea; 4. Intestinal parasitism, stomachache. Use rind 10-15 gm., as decoction. Externally useful in paddyfield dermatitis, scalds. Boil herb in water for washing, or pulverize and use as poultice.

Prescriptions　　1. Chronic diarrhea: Rind of Punica granatum 15 gm., Myristica fragrans 10 gm., as decoction.

2. Chronic dysentery: Rind of Punica granatum. Pulsatilla chinensis, Portulaca oleracea, Plantago major, 15 gm. each, as decoction.

3. Tape worm and ascaris infestation: Grind Punica granatum rind and betel nuts into fine powder, take 5 gm. twice daily for two days.

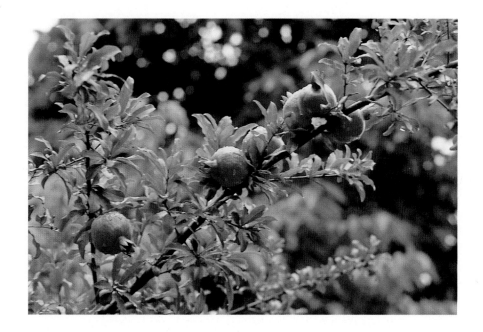

　　石榴科、石榴屬之落葉灌木或小喬木，高可達7米。嫩莖常呈四稜形，較軟弱，莖頂常演變成刺狀。葉對生或近簇生，長矩圓形或長倒卵形，中脈在葉背凸起。花1至數朵生於枝頂或腋生，有短梗；花萼鐘形，紅色，質厚，質端 5 至 7 裂；花瓣與萼片同數，生於萼筒內，稍高出於萼片，紅色，偶有白色；雄蕊多數，花絲細弱；子房下位，中軸胎座。漿果近球形，果肉紅色多汁。種子多數。花期：夏季。

Punicaceae: Deciduous shrubs or small trees, up to 7m high. Young stems usually 4 ridged, weak, tips modified into thorns. Leaves opposite or fasciculate, oblong or oblong-obovate, mid-rib raised beneath. Flowers one or several, borne in axils or terminally, pedicels short; calyx campanulate, red, thick, 5-7 lobed; petals red or occasionally white, equal sepals in number, borne inside the calyx tube, slightly exceeding the sepals, stamens numerous, filaments delicate; ovary inferior, placenta axile. Berries subglobose, pulp red and juicy. Seeds numerous. Flowering in summer.

大 羅 傘 樹

Ardisia hanceana Mez

別　　名　　漢斯紫金牛、大羅傘。

生長環境　　生於林下陰濕地。

採集加工　　藥用根、葉。切片、曬乾或鮮用。

性味功能　　味辛、苦，性平。解毒，活血，祛風濕。

主治用法　　1. 咽喉腫痛，目赤腫痛；2. 風濕痹痛，肢體麻木。每用 3 至 4 錢，水煎服。外用治跌打損傷，適量鮮葉、根，搗爛敷患處。

附　　註　　華東地區有將本品代替朱砂根（Ardisia crenata）入藥。

Habitat　　On damp soil under woods.

Preparation　　Use roots and leaves, slice, dry under sun or use fresh.

Properties　　Acrid and bitter tasting; neutral. Anti-inflammatory; promotes circulation; anti-rheumatic.

Indications　　1. Sore throat, sore eyes; 2. Rheumatic pains, numbness of extremities. Use 10-12 gm., as decoction. External use in traumatic injury, mash suitable quantity of leaves and roots for use as poultice.

Remarks　　In eastern China, this is used in place of Ardisia crenata in prescriptions.

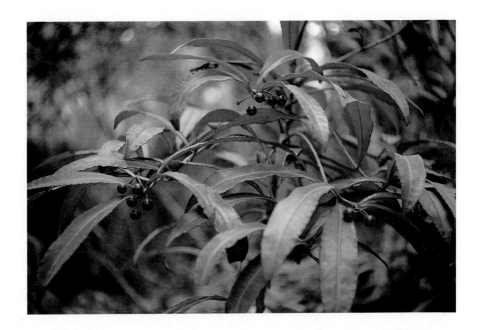

　　紫金牛科、紫金牛屬之灌木。莖粗壯，無分枝，但有側生之特殊花枝。葉堅紙質，橢圓狀或長圓狀披針形，近全緣或具邊緣反捲的疏鋸齒、齒尖有腺點，葉背近葉緣處具稀疏隆起之腺點。複傘房狀傘形花序，着生於頂端下彎之側生特殊花枝之尾端；花萼基部連合，萼片卵形，具少量腺點；花瓣白色或帶紫色，具腺點；花藥箭狀披針形，背有大腺點；花瓣、雄蕊、雌蕊等長。花期：七月。

　　Myrsinaceae: Shrubs. Stem strong, unbranched, but with modified lateral floral shoots. Leaves firm papery, elliptic or oblong-lanceolate, subentire or margins with distanced reflexed teeth, tips of teeth glandular, raised glands sparsely spaced along the margins beneath. Compound corymbose umbels at the tips of drooping lateral floral shoots; calyx united at base, sepals ovate, with a few glandular marks; petals white or whitish-purple, punctate; anthers sagittate lanceolate, with large glandular spots at back; petals, stamens and pistils similar in length. Flowering in July.

虎 舌 紅

Ardisia mamillata Hance

別　　名　紅毛氈、紅毛走馬胎、紅毛紫金牛。

生長環境　生於山谷、林下陰濕處。

採集加工　藥用全株。夏末秋初採摘，切片，曬乾或鮮用。

性味功能　味苦、微辛，性涼。清熱利濕，活血止血。

主治用法　1. 風濕痺痛，跌打損傷；2. 肺結核咳血；3. 血滯經閉，痛經；4. 肝炎，膽囊炎。每用3至5錢，水煎服。孕婦忌服。癰瘡腫毒，葉外用適量搗敷。

方　　例　1. 風濕痺痛：虎舌紅1兩，水、黃酒各半煎服。

2. 血滯經閉，痛經：虎舌紅、雞血藤、香附子各4錢，水煎服。

3. 跌打損傷：虎舌紅1兩，浸白酒500毫升，七天後，每次服10毫升，每日3次。

Habitat　　In ravines, under woods in damp shady places.

Preparation　　Use whole herb. Collect at end of summer and early autumn, slice, dry under sun or use fresh.

Properties　　Bitter and slightly acrid tasting; cold. Anti-inflammatory, anti-rheumatic; promotes circulation; haemostatic.

Indications　　Rheumatism, traumatic injury; 2. Pulmonary tuberculosis with haemoptysis; 3. Amenorrhea, dysmenorrhea; 4. Hepatitis, cholecystitis. Use 10-15 gm., as decoction. Contraindicated in pregnancy. For boils and abscesses, mash fresh herb and use as poultice.

Prescriptions　　1. Rheumatism: Ardisia mamillata 30 gm., boil with equal amounts of wine and water as decoction.

2. Amenorrhea, dysmenorrhea: Ardisia mamillata, Millettia reticulata, Cyperus rotundus rhizomes, 12 gm. each, as decoction.

3. Traumatic injury: Ardisia mamillata 30 gm., steep in white wine 500ml for 7 days, then consume the wine 10 ml. each time, 3 times daily.

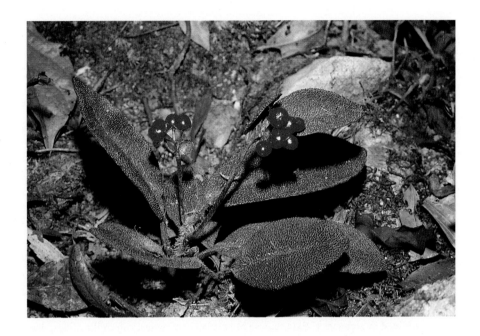

　　紫金牛科、紫金牛屬之半灌木，高約20厘米。具匍匐木質根狀莖，嫩莖有褐色捲縮分節毛。葉互生，紙質，橢圓形至倒卵形，頂端鈍或急尖，葉緣有不清晰之圓齒，兩面均有腺點及褐色捲縮分節毛，葉面之毛出自疣狀凸起。傘形花序腋生，有花7至15朵，具捲縮分節毛；萼片稍長於花瓣，具黑腺點及捲縮分節毛；花瓣卵形；與子房均有黑腺點。果有黑腺點及毛，成熟時鮮紅色。花期：六月至七月。

　　Myrisinaceae: Subshrubs, up to 20 cm high. Creeping rhizomes woody, young stem with brown curly articulated hairs. Leaves alternate, chartaceous, elliptic or obovate, apex obtuse or acute, margins inconspicuously crenulate, both surfaces punctate and with brown curly articulated hairs, hairs on top surface arising from tuberculate bases. Flowers 7-15, in axillary umbels, with curly articulated hairs; sepals slightly longer than petals, with black glands and curly articulated hairs; petals ovate, and, together with ovary, punctate. Fruits with black glands and hairs, scarlet at maturity. Flowering from June to July.

落地紫金牛

Ardisia primulaefolia Gardn. et Champ.

別　　名　蓮座紫金牛、落地金牛、毛蟲藥。

生長環境　生於山坡林下陰濕地。

採集加工　藥用全株。全年可採，切段，曬乾或鮮用。

性味功能　味苦、微辛，性涼。清熱，活血，止血。

主治用法　1.肺結核咳嗽，咳血；2.便血，痢疾；3.崩漏，痛經；4.風濕痹痛，跌打損傷。每用3至5錢，水煎服。孕婦忌服。瘡癤腫毒，毛蟲刺傷，外用鮮品適量搗敷患處，或煎水外洗。

附　　註　海南島白沙地區，民間用本品毒殺野豬。

Habitat　　On slopes, under woods, and in damp, shaded areas.

Preparation　　Use whole herb. Collect all year round, cut into segments, dry under sun or use fresh.

Properties　　Bitter and slightly acrid tasting; cold. Anti-inflammatory; promotes circulation; haemostatic.

Indications　　Pulmonary tuberculosis with cough, haemoptysis; 2. Melena, dysentery; 3. Uterine bleeding, dysmenorrhea; 4. Rheumatism, traumatic injury. Use 10-15 gm., as decoction. Contraindicated in pregnancy. External use in boils and abscesses, caterpillar stings, mash fresh herb for use as poultice, or boil in water for washing.

Remarks　　In Hainan, this herb is used to poison wild boars.

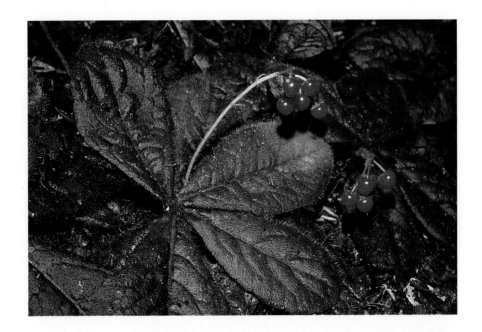

紫金牛科、紫金牛屬之半灌木。近於無莖。葉蓮座狀，膜質；橢圓形至矩圓狀橢圓形，葉頂端圓形或極鈍；葉緣具波狀圓齒及腺點；葉面及背均有捲縮分節之褐色毛，葉背具腺點。傘形或複傘形花序頂生，生於蓮座葉中央，總花梗頂端具1至4叢粉紅斑點小花；萼片卵狀披針形，外面有少數腺點及稀疏捲縮分節毛；花瓣卵形，長與萼片幾相等；花藥背面有腺點。果直徑約6毫米。花期：五月至六月。

Myrsinaceae: Subshrubs, acaulescent. Leaves in a spreading rosette, membranous; elliptic or oblong-elliptic, tip rounded or extremely obtuse; margin wavy, crenulate and punctate; curly brown hairs on both surfaces, punctate beneath. Inflorescences terminal, umbels or compound umbels, bearing at the top one to four clusters of pink spotted flowers; sepals ovate-lanceolate, with sparse glands and curly articulated hairs; petals ovate, similar to sepals in length; anthers punctate at dorsal side. Fruits 6 mm in diameter. Flowering from May to June.

白花酸藤果

Embelia ribes Burm. f.

別　　名　入地龍、水林果、鹹酸藤、酸味藤、喪間。

生長環境　生於山坡、路邊陽光充足處。

採集加工　藥用根、葉。全年可採，根切片曬乾，葉多鮮用。

性味功能　味甘、酸，性平。消炎，止瀉。

主治用法　1. 急性胃腸炎，痢疾；2. 外傷出血，蛇咬傷。每用根 3 至 5 錢，水煎服。葉外用治小兒頭瘡，跌打損傷。鮮葉適量，煎水外洗患處。

主要成分　含蒽醌類、信筒子醌、酸金牛醌。本品所含酸金牛醌鈉鹽，有驅豬蛔蟲、馬蛔蟲、馬蟯蟲的功能，但有引起胃腸炎的副作用。果實含信筒子醌（embelin）及威蘭精（villangin），其提取物對老鼠有避孕和抗生育作用。

Habitat　　On sunny slopes and on roadside.

Preparation　　Use roots and leaves. Collect all year round, slice roots and dry under sun, use leaves fresh.

Properties　　Sweet and sour tasting; neutral. Anti-inflammatory, anti-diarrheal.

Indications　　1. Acute gastro-interitis, dysentery; 2. Wound bleeding, snake bites. Use roots 10-15 gm., as decoction. Leaves are useful for scalp furunculosis of children and for external injury. Boil suitable quantity of fresh leaves in water for washing.

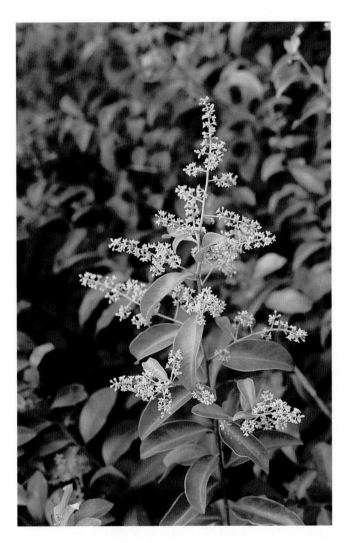

紫金牛科、酸藤果屬之攀援性
灌木。葉互生；矩圓狀橢圓形、橢
圓形或卵形；紙質或堅紙質；葉頂
端漸尖；葉緣略向裏彎；側脈不明
顯。雌雄同株異花；花序圓錐狀，
頂生，多少有葉，有總狀的枝，具
褐色毛；花細小，5出，少有4出；
萼片三角形，有睫毛，花冠裂片分
離，外面被稀疏柔毛，內面及邊緣
有密毛；雄蕊着生於花冠裂片之中
部；雌花柱頭頭狀。果球形，皺
縮。花期：一月至七月。

Myrsinaceae: Climbing shrubs.
Leaves alternate; oblong-elliptic, elliptic
or ovate; chartaceous or firm
chartaceous; apex acuminate; margin
slightly recurved; lateral veins
inconspicuous, Flowers unisexual,
monoecious, panicles terminal, with
some leaves, branches racemous, with
brown hairs; flowers small, 5-merous,
rarely 4-merous; sepals deltoid, with
ciliate hairs; corolla lobes separate,
sparsely villose outside, densely villose
inside and along the margins; stamens
arising at the centre of the corolla lobes;
stigmas capitate. Fruits globose,
wrinkled. Flowering from January to
July.

柿

Diospyros kaki L. f.

別　　名　朱果、柿子、柿樹、柿蒂。

生長環境　多為栽培。

採集加工　藥用全株。根全年可採，葉夏、秋採，果秋、冬採，收集果蒂，曬乾。果加工製成柿餅，柿霜從柿餅上收集。

性味功能　果：味甘，性寒。清熱止血，潤肺生津。柿蒂：味苦，性平。降氣，止呃。柿霜：味甘，性涼。清熱生津。根：味苦、澀，性涼。清熱止血。葉：味苦、酸、澀，性涼。止血，降壓。

主治用法　果：肺燥咳嗽，咽喉乾痛，胃腸出血，痔血，高血壓。柿蒂：呃逆，夜尿。柿霜：咽喉乾痛，聲嘶，口瘡。根：吐血，痔血，血崩。葉：血小板減少性紫癜，功能性子宮出血，潰瘍病出血，咯血，痔血，高血壓。每用柿1至2個，柿蒂、柿霜1至3錢，根2至3錢，水煎服；葉研粉每服1錢。

附　　註　柿嫩葉可作茶劑，作冠心病患者或老年人飲料。

Habitat　　　　Mostly cultivated (as persimmon).

Preparation　　Use whole herb. Collect roots all year round, leaves in summer and autumn, fruits in autumn and winter. Collect fruit stalks and dry under sun. Fruits could be processed into pressed persimmon cakes. Frosting is collected from the pressed persimmon cakes.

Properties　　Fruits: Sweet tasting; cold. Anti-inflammatory, haemostatic; promotes salivary secretion. Fruit stalks: Bitter tasting; neutral. Relieves hiccups. Roots: Bitter and astringent tasting; cool. Anti-inflammatory, haemostatic. Leaves: Bitter, sour and astringent tasting; cool. Haemostatic, hypotensive.

Indications　　Fruits: Dry coughs, sorethroat, gastrointestinal bleeding, haemorrhoidal bleeding, hypertension. Fruit stalks: Hiccups, night frequency. Roots: Haemoptysis, bleeding haemorrhoids, uterine bleeding. Leaves: Thrombocytopenic purpura, functional uterine bleeding, bleeding peptic ulcer, haemoptysis, bleeding haemorrhoids, hypertension. Use fruits 1-2, fruit stalks and frosting 3-10 gm., roots 5-10 gm., as decoction. Leaves are pulverized and taken 3 gm. each time.

Remarks　　　The young, tender leaves of Diospyros kaki are used as tea in coronary artery insufficiency and for old age.

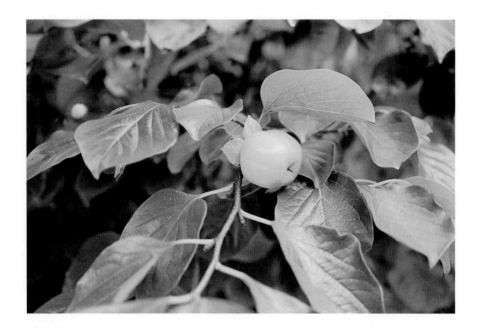

　　柿科、柿樹屬之喬木，高可達15米，樹皮鱗片狀開裂。葉互生，葉片橢圓狀卵形、矩圓狀卵形或倒卵形，長6至18厘米，寬3至9厘米；葉頂端小尖頭，葉基部寬楔形或近圓形；葉背淡綠色，有褐色柔毛；葉柄有毛。花雌雄異株或同株，雄花成短聚傘，雌花單生於葉腋；花萼4深裂，果成熟時萼增大；花冠白色，4裂，有毛。漿果卵圓形或扁球形，橙黃色或鮮黃色，花萼宿存。花期：夏初。

Ebenaceae: Trees, up to 15m high, bark cracked as scales. Leaves alternate, elliptic-ovate, oblong-ovate or obovate, 6-18cm long, 3-9cm broad; apex mucronate, base broad cuneate or suborbicular; light green and brown villose beneath; petioles hairy. Dioecious or monoecious, staminates in short cymes, pistillates solitary and axillary; calyx deeply 4-lobed, enlarged at maturity of fruit; corolla white, 4-lobed, hairy. Berries ovoid or compressed globose, orange or bright yellow, calyx persistent. Flowering in early summer.

白　檀

Symplocos paniculata (Thunb.) Miq.

別　　名　碎米子樹、鳥子樹、臭柴蒲、地胡椒。

生長環境　生於向陽山坡灌木叢中。

採集加工　葉用根或全株。全年可採，曬乾。

性味功能　味苦、澀，性微寒。清熱解毒。

主治用法　1.胃炎，胃腫瘤；2.乳腺炎，瘡癤；3.過敏性皮炎，蕁麻疹。每用根1至2兩，水煎服。外用全株適量，水煎洗患處。

方　　例　胃炎：白檀根、豬瘦肉各1兩5錢，同燉，服湯食肉。

Habitat　　　In thickets along sunny slopes.

Preparation　　Use roots or whole herb. Collect all year round, dry under sun.

Properties　　Bitter and astringent tasting; slightly cold. Anti-inflammatory.

Indications　　1. Gastritis, gastric tumour; 2. Mastitis, furunculosis; 3. Allergic dermatitis, urticaria. Use roots 30-60 gm., as decoction. For external use, boil whole herb in water for washing lesions.

Prescription　　Gastritis: Symplocos paniculata and lean pork, 50 gm. each, boil and consume as food.

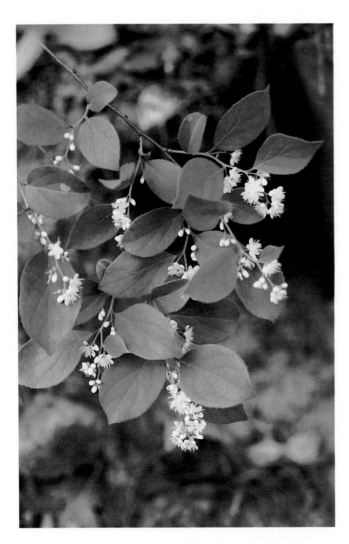

　　山礬科、山礬屬之落葉灌木或小喬木。嫩莖、葉片、葉柄及花序均被柔毛。葉互生，橢圓形或倒卵形，先端急尖或漸尖，葉基楔形，葉緣具細鋸齒，葉面之中脈凹陷。圓錐花序生於新枝之頂端，有長花梗；花萼裂片有睫毛；花冠芳香，5深裂，有極短之花冠筒；雄蕊約30枚，花絲基部合生成五體雄蕊；子房頂端圓錐狀。核果藍色，卵形，稍偏斜，宿存之萼裂片直立。花期：四月至五月。

Symplocaceae: Deciduous shrubs or small trees. Twigs, laminae, petioles and inflorescence all pilose. Leaves alternate, elliptic or obovate, apex acute or acuminate, base cuneiform, margin serrulate, mid-rib impressed on the upper surface. Flowers fragrant, in panicles at end of new branches, pedicels long, calyx lobes ciliate; corolla white, deeply 5-lobed, on an extremely short corolla tube; stamens about 30, filaments united at base to form a pentadelphous (five-bodied) stamen. Fruits drupes, blue, ovoid, conical at the top, slightly skewed, with erect persistent sepals. Flowering from April to May.

桂　花

Osmanthus fragrans Lour.

別　　名　木犀、丹桂、山桂花、銀桂。

生長環境　多為栽培。

採集加工　藥用花、果實及根。秋季採花，冬季採果，四季採根，曬乾用。

性味功能　花：味辛，性溫。散寒破結，化痰止咳。果：味辛、甘，性溫。健胃。根：味甘、微澀，性平。祛風濕。

主治用法　花：牙痛，咳喘痰多，經閉腹痛。果：虛寒胃痛。根：風濕筋骨痛，腰痛，牙痛。每用花、果2至4錢，根2至3兩，水煎服。

方　　例　1.經閉腹痛：桂花1兩，荔枝肉適量，同煮，以紅糖、黃酒沖服。

2.胃痛：桂花果實1錢5分，水煎服；或曬乾研末，每次用1至2分沖服。

3.風濕筋骨痛：桂花根5錢至1兩，水煎服。

主要成分　花含芳香物質，如γ-葵酸內酯，α-紫羅蘭酮（α-ionone）等。

附　　註　桂花可作食品原料，製成桂花糕、桂花糖、桂花茶、桂花酒等。

Habitat　　　Mostly cultivated.

Preparation　　Use flowers, fruits, and roots. Collect flowers in autumn, fruits in winter, roots all year round. Dry under sun.

Properties　　Flowers: Acrid tasting; warm. Expectorant and antitussive. Fruits: Acrid and sweet tasting; warm. Stomachic. Roots: Sweet and slightly astringent tasting; neutral. Anti-rheumatic.

Indications　　Flowers: Toothache, productive cough, amenorrhea and stomachache. Fruits: Gastric discomfort. Roots: Rheumatism, low back pain, toothache. Use flowers and fruits 5-10 gm., roots 60-90 gm., as decoction.

Prescriptions　1. Amenorrhea and stomachache: Osmanthus fragrans flowers 30 gm., boil with suitable quantity of lychee fruits, add yellow sugar, and take with wine.

2. Gastric pain: Osmanthus fragrans fruits 5 gm., as decoction. These could also be dried under sun, ground into powder, and taken 0.3 to 0.5 gm. each time.

3. Rheumatism: Osmanthus fragrans roots 15-30 gm., as decoction.

Remarks　　The flowers of Osmanthus are also used widely in the food industry, where they are incorporated into cakes and confectionery, tea, and wine.

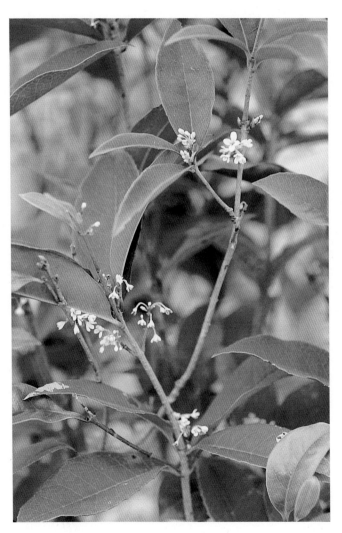

　　木犀科、木犀屬之常綠灌木或小喬木，高約 3 米。樹皮灰色。葉密集生於莖上端，對生，革質，橢圓形至橢圓狀披針形；全緣，或近葉尖之葉緣疏生細鋸齒；葉面主脈常呈淺綠色下凹，於葉背隆起。花序簇生於葉腋，嫩莖、老莖均可見花，花白色至淡黃色，極香；花梗纖細，致花常下垂；花萼 4 裂；花冠筒 4 裂，花瓣橢圓形而稍厚；雄蕊 2，花絲極短，着生於花冠筒近頂部。核果橢圓形，熟時紫黑色。花期：秋季。

Oleaceae: Evergreen shrubs or small trees, up to 3m high, bark greyish. Leaves opposite, coriaceous, densely crowded at ends of branches; elliptic to elliptic-lanceolate; entire or occasionally serrate in the upper half; midrib light green; impressed, raised beneath. Flowers white to light yellow, very fragrant, pedicels delicate, causing the flowers to nod; calyx 4-lobed; corolla tube 4-lobed, petals elliptic; stamens 2, filaments very short, borne near the top of the corolla tube. Drupe ellipsoidal, dark purple when ripe. Flowering in autumn.

109

酸 葉 膠 藤

Ecdysanthera rosea Hook. et Arn.

別　　名　乳藤、酸藤木、紅背酸藤、斑鳩藤、頭林沁、黑風藤。

生長環境　生於山地灌木林中。

採集加工　藥用全株。全年可採，曬乾或鮮用。

性味功能　味酸、微澀，性涼。有毒。利尿，消腫，止痛。

主治用法　1.咽喉腫痛；2.腸炎；3.風濕骨痛。每用5錢至1兩，水煎服。孕婦忌服。外用治跌打瘀腫，疔瘡。鮮葉適量，煎水外洗，搗爛敷患處。

主要成分　葉含游離酒石酸 1.7%，酒石酸鉀約 5%。莖乳汁中含多量橡膠。

Habitat　On hills and thickets.

Preparation　Use whole herb. Collect all year round. Dry under sun or use fresh.

Properties　Sour and slightly astringent tasting; cool. Toxic, diuretic, anti-swelling, analgesic.

Indicatios　1. Sore throat; 2. Enteritis; 3. Rheumatic bone pain. Use 15-30 gm., as decoction. Contraindicated in pregnancy. External use in traumatic bruises, furuncles. Boil fresh leaves in water for washing, or use as poultice.

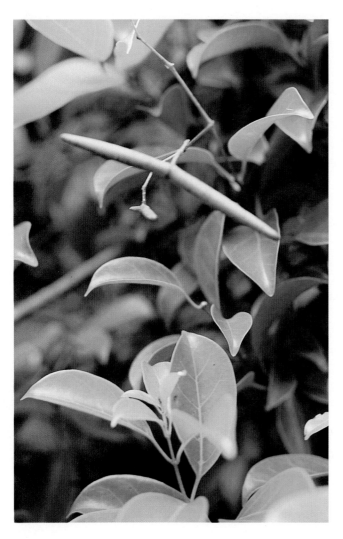

夾竹桃科、花皮膠藤屬之木質大型藤本，長可達 10 米。莖深褐色，枝條上部淡綠色，有乳汁。葉對生、紙質，寬橢圓形，長 3 至 7 厘米，葉背有白粉；側脈每邊 4 至 6 條。聚傘花序圓錐狀廣開展，3 歧，總花梗略有白色粉及短柔毛；花萼 5 深裂，內基部有腺體；花冠粉紅色，近罎狀，花瓣 5 片，向右覆蓋；雄蕊 5 枚，着生於花冠筒之基部；花盤環狀；心皮離生。蓇葖果雙生，有明顯斑點。種子頂端有種毛。花期：四月至十二月。

Apocynaceae: Large lactiferous lianas climbing over trees, up to 10m high; stem dark purple, branchlets green. Leaves opposite, papery, broad elliptic, 3-7 cm long, glaucous beneath; lateral nerves 4-6 on each side. Flowers small, white pink, in terminal corymbose panicles, trichotomous, peduncle glaucous and pilose; calyx 5-parted, inside glandular; corolla suburceolate, petals 5, turning to the right; stamens 5, inserted to the base of corolla tube; disc annular; carpels 2, separate. Follicles paired, spotted. Seeds comose. Flowering from April to December.

白 葉 藤

Cryptolepis sinensis (Lour.) Merr.

別　　名　紅藤仔、脫皮藤、飛揚藤、牛蹄藤。

生長環境　生於山坡、水溝邊。

採集加工　藥用全株。全年可採，曬乾或鮮用。

性味功能　味甘、淡，性涼。有小毒。清熱解毒，止血，止痛。

主治用法　1.肺熱咳血；2.胃潰瘍出血。每用鮮品3至5錢，水煎服。外用治毒蟲、蛇咬傷，疥瘡，瘡毒潰瘍，跌打刀傷，鮮品搗敷患處。

方　　例　1.肺熱咳血，胃潰瘍出血：白葉藤鮮品半斤，搗爛取汁，蜜糖適量沖服。另取莖葉2兩，水煎服，每日1至2劑。

2.毒蟲、蛇咬傷，瘡毒潰瘍：白葉藤鮮品3至5錢，搗汁沖酒服，並外用鮮品搗敷患處。

附　　註　本品服用過量，會有腹痛等副作用。

Habitat　　On slopes, along gullies.

Preparation　　Use whole herb. Collect all year round, dry under sun or use fresh.

Properties　　Sweet, bland tasting; cool. Slightly poisonous, anti-inflammatory, haemostatic, analgesic.

Indications　　1. Haemoptysis; 2. Gastric ulcer bleeding. Use fresh herb 10-15 gm., as decoction. External use in insect and snake bites, scabies, boils, ulcer, knife wound, by applying mashed herb to lesions.

Prescriptions　　1. Haemoptysis, gastric ulcer bleeding: Fresh Cryptolepis sinensis 1/2 catty (300 gm.), mash to extract juice, mix with honey for oral use. Also use 60 gm. of leaves and stem as decoction, take once or twice daily.

2. Insect and snake bites, boils and ulcer: Fresh Cryptolepis sinensis 10-15 gm., extract juice and mix with wine for oral use, also apply mashed fresh herb to the lesion.

Remarks　　Overdose may result in stomachache.

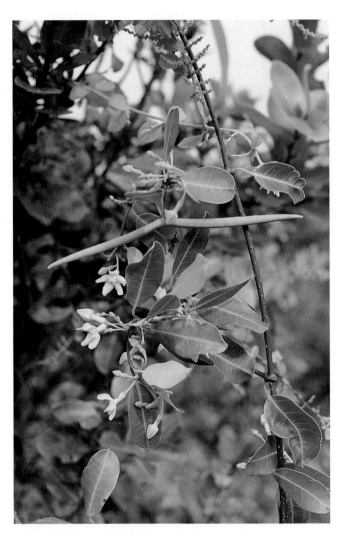

蘿藦科、白葉藤屬之多年生木質藤本。以右旋方式纏繞於其他物體之上，具乳汁。嫩莖通常為紅褐色。葉對生，矩圓形；頂端圓形而具小尖頭，葉基近圓形；葉面深綠色，葉背蒼白色。聚傘花序頂生或腋生；花蕾矩圓形，頂端尾狀漸尖；花萼 5 裂，內方有腺體 10 枚；花冠淡黃色，花瓣條狀披針形，且比花冠筒長兩倍，向右覆蓋；副花冠生於花冠筒內面；雄蕊 5 枚，載粉器匙形。菁葖果長披針形。種子頂端具白色絹質種毛。花期：四月至九月。

Asclepiadaceae: Perennial woody vines, twining on other objects in a right-handed fashion, lactiferous. Young stems maroon. Leaves opposite, oblong; apex rounded and apiculate, base suborbicular; upper surface dark green, lower surface pale. Flowers in axillary or terminal cymes; flower buds oblong, tip caudate acuminate; sepals 5, with 10 glands on the inside; corolla light yellow, petals linear-lanceolate, twice the length of corolla tube, imbricating on the right, corona a rising inside the corolla tube; stamens 5, "translator" or arm spatulate. Follicles long lanceolate. Tip of seeds with a coma of white silky hairs. Flowering from April to September.

天 星 藤

Graphistemma pictum (Champ.) Benth. et Hook. f. ex Maxim.

別　　名　　大奶藤、牛奶藤、雞腿果、羅摩藤。

生長環境　　生於路邊灌木林中。

採集加工　　藥用全株。全年可採，曬乾或鮮用。

性味功能　　味辛，性溫。催乳，活血。

主治用法　　1.乳汁不足；2.喉痛；3.跌打損傷，骨折。每用1至3錢，水煎服。
外用鮮品適量，搗爛敷患處。

Habitat	Among roadside bushes.
Preparation	Use whole herb. Collect all year round, dry under sun or use fresh.
Properties	Acrid tasting; warm. Galactogogue; promotes circulation.
Indications	1. Insufficient breast milk secretion; 2. Sore throat; 3. Traumatic injury,

fractures. Use 3-10 gm., as decoction. Mash fresh herb for external use as poultice.

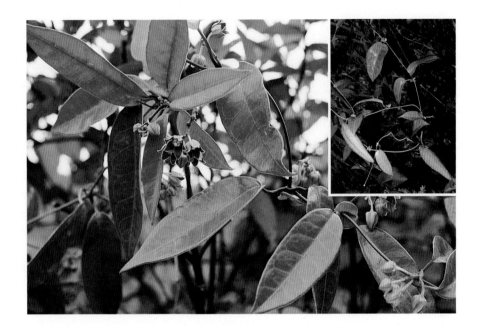

蘿藦科、天星藤屬之多年生木質右旋藤本，植株具豐富乳汁。葉對生，矩圓形，葉尖呈漸尖，葉基圓形；葉柄頂端叢生小腺體；托葉葉狀，脈紋明顯。總狀式聚傘花序腋生；花萼5裂，內面基部有腺體；花冠外面綠色，內面深紫紅色，有黃色邊。果大型，木質，披針形，似羊角形。種子具膜狀翅，頂端有降落傘狀白色種毛，毛長約4厘米。花期：六月至七月。

Asclepiadaceae: Lactiferous perennial woody vines with a right-handed twining. Leaves opposite, oblong; apex acuminate, base round; cluster of small glands on the upper part of the petioles; stipules leaf-like; veins prominent. Cymose racemes axillary; calyx segments 5, internal base punctate; corolla greenish outside, deep purple-scarlet inside; margin yellowish. Fruits large, woody, lanceolate, horn-like. Seeds with membranous wings, apex attached with white parachute-like hairs which are about 4cm long. Flowering from June to July.

月 光 花

Calonyction aculeatum (L.) House

別　　名　天茄兒、嫦娥奔月。

生長環境　多栽培作觀賞，或逸生於路邊。

採集加工　藥用全株及種子。夏、秋採收，多為鮮用。

主治用法　全株：治蛇傷。種子：治跌打腫痛，骨折。骨折復位後，外用鮮品搗敷患處。本品肉質萼及嫩葉可作蔬菜，乾花可做湯及點心。

附　　註　本品可用於嫁接番薯，增加產量。

Habitat　　　Mostly cultivated, or having escaped and growing wild along roadside.

Preparation　　Use whole herb and seeds. Collect in summer and autumn, use fresh.

Indications　　Whole herb: Snake bites. Seeds: Traumatic injury, fractures. After repositioning fractures, apply mashed fresh herb as poultice. The young leaves and the fleshy calyces of the flowers are edible as vegetables. The dried flowers are used in soups and tidbits ("dim sum").

Remarks　　This herb when used as stock for the grafting of Ipomoea batatas (sweet potato) will lead to increased yield.

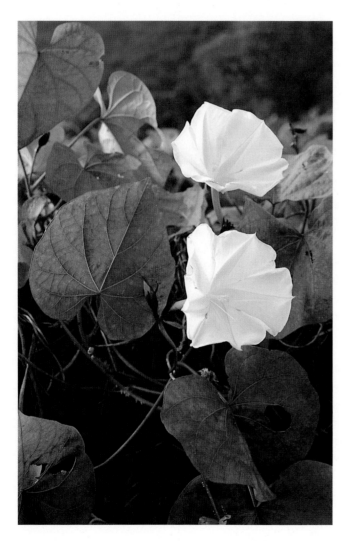

旋花科、月光花屬之一年生右旋纏繞草本，長可達 10 米。莖有乳汁，綠色，近平滑或具少量軟刺。葉卵形，全緣或稍有角或分裂；葉頂端長銳尖或漸尖，葉基心形。花大朵，芳香，夜間開放；1 至多朵排列成總狀，有時循軸 "之" 字曲折；萼片卵形，有長芒，花冠大，雪白色，極美麗，瓣中帶淡綠色；雄蕊及雌蕊伸出花外；雄蕊 5，花藥淡黃色；花盤環狀，厚肉質。蒴果具銳尖頭，果柄粗厚。花期：四月至十一月。

Convolvulaceae: Annual right-handed twining herbs, up to 10m long; stem lactiferous, green, nearly smooth or with a few soft spines. Leaves ovate, entire, slightly angular, or shallowly lobed; apex acute or acuminate, base cordate. Flowers large, fragrant, blooming at night, 1 to several in a raceme, or sometimes in a zigzag arrangement along the rachis; sepals ovate, possessing a long awn; corolla large, white, showy, petals carrying a light tinge of green; stamens and pistils extending beyond the flower; stamens 5, anthers light yellow; floral-disc annular, succulent. Capsules with a pointed head, stalk stout. Flowering from April to November.

菟 絲 子

Cuscuta australis R. Br.

別　　名　無娘藤、無根草、金綫草、黃絲、狐絲。

生長環境　生於路旁草叢、溝邊等地。

採集加工　藥用種子。秋季果實成熟時採收，打下種子，曬乾。

性味功能　味甘，性溫。補肝腎，益精，明目，安胎。

主治用法　1. 腎虛，腰膝酸軟，頭暈目眩；2. 陽痿，遺精；3. 遺尿，尿頻，尿有餘瀝；4. 視力減退，耳鳴；5. 習慣性流產，胎動不安。每用 2 至 4 錢，水煎服。外用治白癜風。

方　　例　1. 男子精氣虧損，中年無子：古方「五子衍宗丸」：菟絲子、五味子、覆盤子、車前子、沙苑蒺藜子各 3 錢，水煎服，或研末為丸服。

2. 習慣性流產：菟絲子、桑寄生、續斷各 3 錢，水煎服。

主要成分　種子含膽甾醇（cholesterol）、菜油甾醇、β - 谷甾醇、豆甾醇等。

Habitat　　Along roadside bushes, or stream edges.

Preparation　　Use seeds. Collect fruits in autumn when ripe, remove the seeds to dry under sun.

Properties　　Sweet tasting; warm. Tonic to "liver", "spleen"; improve eyesight, stabilize pregnancy.

Indications　　1. Weak "kidney", sore knees, dizziness; 2. Impotence, nocturnal ejaculation; 3. Urinary frequency, enuresis; 4. Failing eyesight, tinnitus; 5. Habitual abortion, fetal distress. Use 5-12 gm., as decoction. External use in cases of vitiligo.

Prescriptions　　1. Weakened masculinity, infertility: Cuscuta australis, Schisandra chinensis fruits, Rubus chingii fruits, Plantago major seeds, Astragalus complanatus seeds, 10 gm. each, as decoction, or pulverize and make into pellets.

2. Habitual abortion: Cuscuta australis, Taxillus chinensis, Dipsacus asper, 10 gm. each, as decoction.

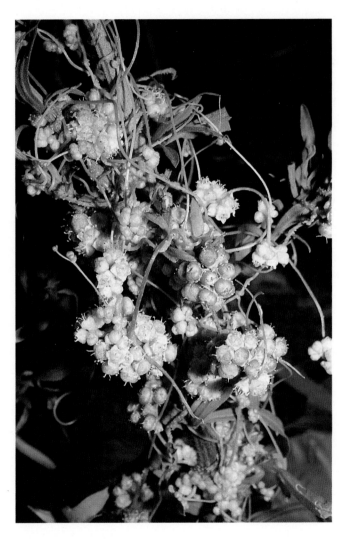

　　旋花科、菟絲子屬之一年生寄生草本。莖幼細，以右旋方式纏繞於其寄主之莖上，黃色，無葉。花多數，簇生；花萼杯狀，5 裂；花冠白色，壺狀或鐘狀；雄蕊 5，花絲短，與花冠裂片互生。本種與田野常見之 C.chinensis 外形及療效極相似。本種宿存花冠只包圍着蒴果之下半部；雄蕊着生於花冠裂片間彎缺處；而後者宿存花冠全包着蒴果；雄蕊着生於花冠裂片間彎缺處之下方。花期：六月至十月。

Convolvulaceae: Annual parasitic herb. Stems yellow, leafless, long and slender, twining over the host in a right-handed fashion, with haustoria penetrating into the host to absorb nutrients. Flowers numerous, in clusters; calyx cupular, 5-lobed; corolla white, urn-shaped or campanulate; stamens 5, filaments short, alternate with the corolla lobes. This herb and C. chinensis are quite similar in appearance as well as therapeutic effects. The fruits of this herb are surrounded by the persistent corolla only to the lower half; stamens arise from the sinus of the corolla lobes; while in the latter case the fruits are almost completely surrounded by the persistent corolla ; stamens arise from below the sinus of the corolla lobes. Flowering from June to October.

土 丁 桂

Evolvulus alsinoides L.

別　　名　白毛將、白鴿草、毛將軍、銀絲草、鹿含草。

生長環境　生於乾旱山坡上。

採集加工　藥用全草。秋季採集，曬乾或鮮用。

性味功能　味苦、澀，性平。止咳平喘，清熱利濕。

主治用法　1. 支氣管哮喘，咳嗽；2. 胃痛，消化不良；3. 腸炎，痢疾；4. 泌尿系感染，白帶；5. 跌打損傷，腰腿痛。每用 3 至 5 錢，水煎服。外用治瘡癤，鮮品適量煎洗或搗敷患處。

方　　例　1. 痢疾：鮮土丁桂 1 至 2 兩，紅糖 5 錢，水煎服，日服 2 次。

2. 白帶：土丁桂 1 兩，銀杏 12 粒，水煎服。

主要成分　含黃酮甙、酚類、氨基酸、糖類、卅烷和 β - 谷甾醇等。

Habitat　　　On dry slopes.

Preparation　Use whole herb. Collect in autumn, dry under sun or use fresh.

Properties　Bitter and astringent tasting; neutral. Antitussive; relieves wheezing; anti-inflammatory, diuretic.

Indications　1. Bronchial asthma, cough; 2. Gastric pain, indigestion; 3. Enteritis, dysentery; 4. Urinary tract infection, leucorrhea; 5. Traumatic injury, knee and back pain. Use 10-15 gm., as decoction. External use in pyodermas, boil fresh herb for washing, or mash herb for local application.

Prescriptions　1. Dysentery: Evolvulus alsinoides 30-60 gm., brown sugar 15 gm., as decoction, to be taken twice daily.

2. Leucorrhea: Evolvulus alsinoides 30 gm., Ginkgo biloba (ginkgo) nuts 12 pieces, as decoction.

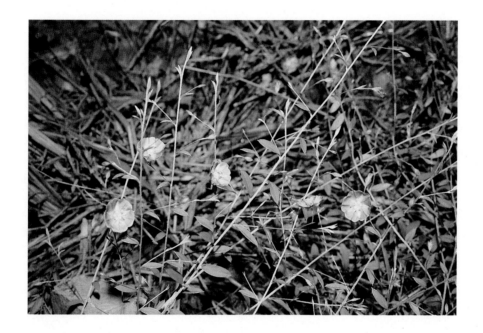

　　旋花科、土丁桂屬之一年生纖細草本。全株被毛，高約50厘米，多分枝，莖直立或斜升。葉互生，葉片卵形，矩圓形或橢圓形，密被毛，全緣，具短柄或幾無柄。花腋生，細小，單生或2至3朵叢生，總花梗纖細而比葉片長得多；苞片2，條形，被毛；萼片5，被長柔毛；花冠漏斗狀，淡藍色或白色，5淺裂；雄蕊5；雌蕊柱頭綫狀或棒狀。蒴果近球形，4瓣開裂。種子4枚。花期：五月至九月。

Convolvulaceae: Annual delicate herbs, pilose throughout, about 50cm high, many branchlets, stems erect or oblique. Leaves alternate, lamina ovate, oblong or elliptic, densely pilose, entire, short-petioled or subsessile. Flowers tinged light blue or white, axillary, small, solitary or 2-3 in a cluster, peduncle delicate and much longer than lamina; bracts 2, linear, hairy; sepals 5, pilose; corolla funnel-shaped, shallowly 5 lobed; stamens 5; stigma linear or clavate. Capsule subglobose, containing 4 seeds, opening by 4 valves. Flowering between May and September.

籬 欄 網

Merremia hederacea (Burm. f.) Hall. f.

別　　名　魚黃草、茉欒藤、小花山豬菜、籬網藤。

生長環境　生於路旁草叢中。

採集加工　藥用全草。夏、秋採收，曬乾或鮮用。

性味功能　味甘、淡，性涼。清熱解毒。

主治用法　1.感冒；2.扁桃體炎，咽喉炎；3.急性眼結膜炎。每用3至5錢，水煎服。外用治瘡癤，適量煎水外洗。種子：研末吹喉，治扁桃體炎。

Habitat　　　Among roadside bushes.

Preparation　Use whole herb. Collect in summer and autumn, dry under sun or use fresh.

Properties　Sweet, bland tasting; cool. Anti-inflammatory.

Indications　1. Influenza; 2. Tonsillitis, sore throat; 3. Acute conjunctivitis. Use 10-15 gm., as decoction. External use for furuncle, boil herb in water for washing. Seeds are ground into powder and blown to throat for treatment of tonsillitis.

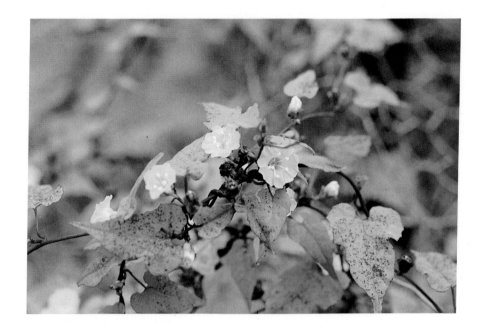

　　旋花科、魚黃草屬之一年生纏繞草本。植株細弱，近光滑，長可達3米。葉互生，掌狀3深裂；葉尖呈漸尖，葉基心形；葉片長2至5厘米。聚傘花序約與葉柄等長，腋生，花3至5朵；萼片5，近卵形；花冠黃色，鐘狀，頂端5淺裂；雄蕊5，不等長；子房上位，花柱長，頭狀柱頭。蒴果卵形，長約6毫米，光滑，有棱。種子4粒。花期：十月至十一月。

Convolvulaceae: Annual twining herbs, delicate, nearly glabrous, up to 3m in length. Leaves alternate, palmately deep 3-lobed, apex acuminate, base cordate; lamina 2-5cm long. Cymes axillary, equalling petioles in length; flowers 3 to 5; sepals 5, near ovate; corolla yellowish, bell shaped, limbs shallowly 5-lobed; stamens 5, unequal; ovary superior, styles long, stigmas capitate. Capsules ovate, 6mm in length, glabrous, with ridges. Seeds 4. Flowering from October to November.

蔦 蘿 松

Quamoclit pennata (Desr.) Boj.

別　　名　蔦蘿、女羅、金鳳毛、翠翎草、錦屏封、金絲綫。

生長環境　多為栽培。

採集加工　藥用全草。夏、秋季採集，多鮮用。

性味功能　味淡，性平。清熱解毒。

主治用法　1.耳疔，瘡癤；2.痢疾，痔血。每用2至3錢，水煎服。外用鮮品煎水洗患處。

Habitat	Mostly cultivated.
Preparation	Use whole herb. Collect in summer and autumn, use fresh.
Properties	Bland tasting; neutral. Anti-inflammtory.
Indications	1. Boils of the ear, pyodermas; 2. Dysentery, bleeding haemorrhoids. Use 5-10 gm., as decoction. For external use, boil herb in water for washing.

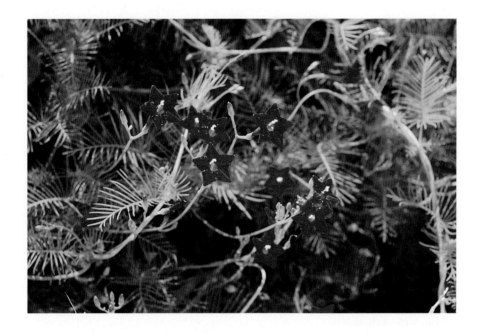

　　旋花科、蒿蘿屬之一年生右旋纏繞性草本。莖柔弱幼細，光滑，嫩莖綠色，莖長度可達4米。葉互生，羽狀細裂，長4至7厘米；裂片幼條形，基部裂片之二裂片再二裂；幼葉之葉柄短，成長葉之葉柄長，葉柄扁平狀；托葉與葉同形狀。聚傘花序腋生，有花數朵，通常較葉長；萼片5；花冠長筒狀，深紅色5裂，筒上部稍膨大；雄蕊5，不等長，外伸。蒴果卵圓形。花期：七月至十月。

Convolvulaceae: Annual right-handed twining herbs. Stems delicate, glabrous, young stems green, up to 4m long. Leaves alternate, finely pinnately lobed, 4-7cm long; pinnae linear, basal pinnae twice divided; young leaves short-petiolate, mature leaves with long petioles, compressed; stipules similar in shape to leaves. Flowers scarlet, several in axillary cymes, inflorescences often longer than leaves; sepals 5; corolla long tubular, swelling above, 5 lobed; stamens 5, of various lengths, extending beyond the corolla tube. Capsules ovoid. Flowering from July to October.

華 石 梓

Gmelina chinensis Benth.

別　　名　石梓、笛籇狗腳迹、鼻血籇。

生長環境　生於山坡、路旁灌木叢中。

採集加工　藥用根。全年可採，切片，曬乾。

性味功能　味甘、微辛、苦，性微溫。有小毒。活血，祛瘀，止痛。

主治用法　1.閉經；2.風濕。每用3至5錢，水煎服。孕婦忌服。

方　　例　1.閉經：華石梓1兩5錢，燉瘦肉服。

2.風濕：華石梓、大羅傘、鷹不泊，均用根，各5錢，水煎服。

Habitat　　On slopes and among roadside bushes.

Preparation　　Use root. Collect all year round, cut into segments. dry under sun.

Properties　　Sweet, acrid, bitter tasting; mildly warm. Slightly toxic. Promotes circulation, resolves bruises, analgesic.

Indications　　1. Amenorrhea; 2. Rheumatism. Use 10-15 gm., as decoction. Contraindicated in pregnancy.

Prescriptions　　1. Amenorrhea: Gmelina chinensis 45 gm., cook with pork for oral use.

2. Rheumatism: Gmelina chinensis, Ardisia crenata, Zanthoxylum avicennae, all using roots, 15 gm. each, as decoction.

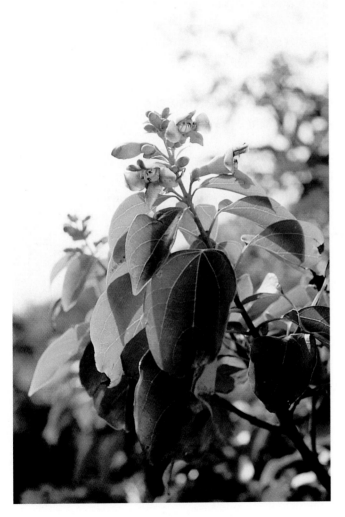

　　馬鞭草科、石梓屬之喬木，高約9米。樹皮栗殼色，枝條上有明顯的皮孔。葉對生，寬卵形至卵狀橢圓形，長5至15厘米，寬6至9厘米，全緣；葉尖呈漸尖，葉基寬楔形至截形；葉面綠色，葉背灰白色。聚傘花序或圓錐花序頂生；苞片葉狀，卵形；花萼鐘狀，頂端截形，裂片有腺點；花冠外面白色，內面淡黃色或淡紫色。果實倒卵形。花期：五月至六月。

Verbenaceae: Trees, 9m high, bark chestnut coloured, lenticels prominent. Leaves opposite, broad-ovate or ovate-elliptic; 5-15cm long, 6-9cm wide; margin entire; acuminate at the apex, base broad-cuneate to truncate; green above, pale beneath. Inflorescence in terminal cymes or panicles, bracts foliaceous, ovate; calyx bell-shaped, truncate at top, lobes possessing glandular spots; corolla whitish outside, pale yellow or pale violet inside. Fruits obovate. Flowering from May to June.

五 指 茄

Solanum mammosum L.

別　　名　　五角茄、五指丁茄、五代同堂、乳茄、北美乳茄。

生長環境　　多為栽培。

採集加工　　藥用果實。秋、冬季果實成熟時採收，多為鮮用。

性味功能　　味苦、澀，性寒。有毒。散瘀消腫。

主治用法　　1.淋巴結炎；2.瘡癤癰腫。外敷患處。

方　　例　　治瘡癤癰腫：五指茄鮮果切為兩半，火烤熱敷患處。

主要成分　　含茄解定（solasodine）、茄解寧（solasodiene）、薯蕷皂甙配基（diosgenin）等。

Habitat	Mostly cultivated.
Preparation	Use fruits. Collect in autumn and winter when fruits ripen. Use fresh.
Properties	Bitter and astringent tasting; cold. Toxic. Reduces swelling and ecchymosis.
Indications	1. lymphadenitis; 2. Carbuncles and furuncles. Apply herb to lesion.
Prescription	Carbuncles and furuncles: Cut fresh fruits of Solanum mammosum into halves, toast warm and apply to lesion.
Remarks	Contains solasodine, solasodiene, and diosgenin.

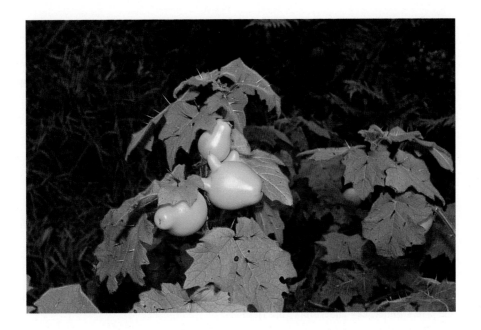

　　茄科、茄屬之直立草本。莖被短柔毛及扁刺，嫩莖被具節之長柔毛、腺毛及扁刺，扁刺蠟黃色而光亮、基部淡紫色、直或略彎。葉圓卵形，長與寬幾相等，通常5裂，裂片淺波狀，兩面密被亮白色極長之柔毛及短柔毛；葉柄具槽、長柔毛、腺毛及皮刺。蝎尾狀花序腋外生，被與枝葉相似之毛，通常3至4朵花；花冠紫槿色，5深裂，外面被長柔毛而內面無毛。漿果土黃色，倒梨狀。花期：夏、秋間。

Solanaceae: Erect herbs. Stems pilose and with flat spines, twigs with articulated villi, glandular hairs and flat spines; spines wax-yellowish and glossy, base tinged purple, straight or slightly curved. Leaves orbicular-ovate, width about equal to length, often 5-lobed with undulate margins, densely covered with long and short white hairs on both sides; petiole grooved, villose with glandular hairs and spines. Flowers 3-4 in axillary scorpioid inflorescence, covered with hairs similar to those on stems and leaves; corolla violet, deeply 5-lobed, villose outside, glabrous inside. Berries mud-yellow in colour, inverted pear-shaped. Flowering between summer and autumn.

茄（矮瓜）

Solanum melongena L.

別　　名　茄子、白茄、紫茄、落蘇。

生長環境　多為栽培。

採集加工　全株入藥。夏、秋採果，秋季植物枯萎時採根，曬乾或鮮用。

性味功能　味甘，性涼。根：清熱利濕，止咳，止血；果：清熱，活血；葉：解毒，消腫。

主治用法　1.風濕性關節炎；2.慢性支氣管炎；3.尿血，便血。每用根5錢至1兩，水煎服。外用治癰瘡癤腫，尋常疣，乳癌潰爛。乾葉研末，或鮮葉搗敷。

方　　例　1.風濕性關節炎，類風濕性關節炎：白茄根5錢，水煎服。或白茄根90克，浸白酒500毫升，三天後開始服，每次服15毫升，每天兩次。

2.癰瘡癤腫：鮮茄子一個焙熱，切開兩側，加煙絲少許，趁熱外敷患處。

主要成分　果實含胡蘆巴鹼、水蘇鹼及茄鹼等多種生物鹼；葉含龍葵鹼等。

附　　註　茄子可供蔬食，民間認為多食恐損目眼矇。

Habitat　　Mostly cultivated (as egg-plants).

Preparation　　Use whole herb. Collect fruits in summer and autumn, roots in autumn when the plants wither. Dry under sun or use fresh.

Properties　　Sweet tasting; cool. Roots: Anti-inflammatory; promote circulation. Leaves: Anti-inflammatory; reduce swelling.

Indications　　1. Rheumatic arthritis; 2. Chronic bronchitis; 3. Haematuria, melena. Use roots, 15-30 gm., as decoction. External use in furuncles, carbuncles, urticaria, and breast cancer ulceration. Pulverize dry leaves, or mash fresh leaves as poultice.

Prescriptions　　1. Rheumatic arthritis, rheumatoid arthritis: Solanum melongena roots 15 gm., as decoction. Also immerse roots 90 gm. in 500 ml. wine for three days, then take 15 ml. twice daily.

2. Furuncles and carbuncles: Toast fresh egg-plant and cut lengthwise, add some tobacco, and apply while hot to lesion.

Remarks　　Egg-plant is mostly consumed as vegetable. There is a folk belief that over consumption could impair the eyesight.

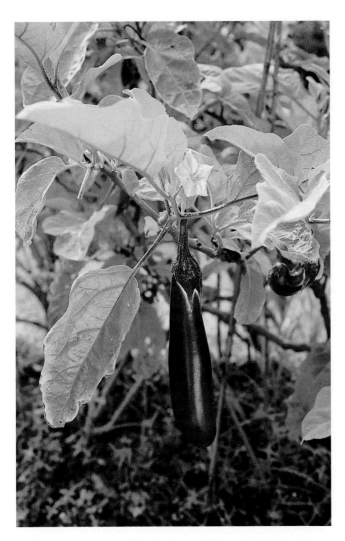

　　茄科、茄屬之直立草本至半灌
木，高可達 1 米。嫩莖、葉、花
梗、花萼均被星狀絨毛。葉卵形至
矩圓狀卵形，葉緣淺波狀至深波狀
圓裂；葉尖鈍形，葉基偏斜。花下
位，花梗短，能孕花單生，花後下
垂；花萼鐘狀，有小皮刺；花冠輻
狀，裂片三角形；雄蕊着生於花冠
筒喉部。漿果較大，圓形或橢圓狀
圓柱形，紫色或白色，萼宿存。花
期：春季至夏季。

Solanaceae: Erect herbs or subshrubs, up to 1m high; young stem,
leaves, pedicels and calyx covered with
stellate woolly hairs. Leaves ovate to
orbicular-ovate, margin undulate to
sinuate; apex obtuse, base oblique.
Flowers hypogynous, pedicels short,
fertile flowers solitary, pendulous after
fertilization; calyx campanulate, spinose;
corolla rotate, segments deltoid; stamens
inserted to the corolla throat. Berries
large, globose or elliptical-cylindrical,
purple or white; calyx persistent.
Flowering from spring to summer.

燈　籠　草

Physalis angulata L.

別　　名　苦蘵、燈籠泡、掛金燈。

生長環境　生於村邊路旁。

採集加工　藥用全草。夏、秋季採集，曬乾或鮮用。

性味功能　味苦，性寒。清熱解毒，利尿。

主治用法　1. 咽喉腫痛，牙齦腫痛；2. 腮腺炎，疱疹。3. 急性肝炎，菌痢。每用 5 錢至 1 兩，水煎服。外用治膿泡瘡，濕疹，適量煎水洗患處。

主要成分　莖葉含酸漿苦味素（physalin）。

Habitat	On roadside along village borders.
Preparation	Use whole herb. Collect in summer and autumn, dry under sun or use fresh.
Properties	Bitter tasting; cold. Anti-inflammatory, diuretic.

Indications　1. Sorethroat, gum pains; 2. Parotitis, herpes zoster. 3. Acute hepatitis, dysentery. Use 15-30 gm., as decoction. Also useful in impetigo and eczema, by boiling herb in water for washing.

Remarks　Leaves and stems contain physalin.

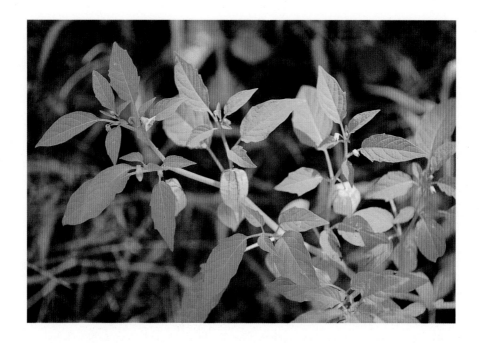

　　茄科、酸漿屬之一年生草本，高30至50厘米，植株被疏短柔毛或近無毛。莖多分枝，分枝纖細。葉互生，或 2 葉雙生於枝的一側，葉片卵形至卵狀橢圓形，全緣或具大小不等之牙齒，葉面及葉背近無毛；葉頂端漸尖或急尖，葉基闊楔形或楔形。花梗纖弱，被短柔毛；花萼鐘狀，5中裂，被短柔毛，果時增大成燈籠狀，完全包圍果實；花冠淡黃色，喉部常有紫色斑紋；花藥藍紫色或有時黃色。果為漿果，種子圓盤狀。花期：五月至十二月。

Solanaceae: Annual herb, 30-50cm high, sparsely pilose or glabrous. Branches much subdivided, twigs slender. Leaves alternate, or appearing as a pair on the same side of the stem, ovate to ovate-elliptic; entire or irregularly toothed, almost glabrous on both sides; apex acuminate or acute, broad cuneiform at base. Pedicel delicate, pilose; sepals bell-shaped, medium 5-lobed, pilose, enlarge on fruiting to completely enclose the fruit; corolla light yellow, often with purple patches at throat; anthers bluish purple or occasionally yellow. Fruit a berry, seeds disk-shaped. Flowering from May to December.

枸 杞 子

Lycium chinense Mill.

別　　名　枸杞、枸杞葉、杞子、地骨皮、甜菜子。

生長環境　多為栽種，或逸生於村邊。

採集加工　藥用果實（杞子）、根皮（地骨皮）、葉。夏、秋季採果實，烘乾。春、秋季採根，剝取根皮，曬乾。春、夏季採葉，多鮮用。

性味功能　果實：味甘，性平。滋補肝腎，益精明目。根皮：味甘，性寒。清熱，涼血，退虛熱。葉：味甘，性平。清熱，明目。

主治用法　果實：1. 精血不足，腰膝酸痛；2. 性神經衰弱；3. 血虛眩暈，視力減退。每用2至4錢，水煎服。根皮：1. 肺結核潮熱；2. 肺熱咳嗽；3. 咯血，衄血。每用3至5錢，水煎服。

方　　例　1. 視力減退：杞子3錢，豬肝適量，蒸熟服。

2. 腎虛腰痛：杞子、金狗脊各4錢，水煎服。

主要成分　果實含甜菜鹼、玉米黃素（zeaxanthin），及多種氨基酸。

附　　註　據《中國藥典》載：枸杞子正品為 L. barbarum。本品功效類似。

Habitat　　Mostly cultivated, or growing along village edges as escapes.

Preparation　　Use fruits, root skins, and leaves. Collect fruits in summer and autumn, roast to dry. Collect roots in spring and autumn, take the skins, dry under sun. Collect leaves in spring and summer, use fresh.

Properties　　Fruits: Sweet tasting; neutral. Tonic to the "liver" and "spleen"; improve eyesight. Root skins: Sweet tasting; neutral. Anti-inflammatory; promote eyesight.

Indications　　Fruits: Oligospermia, knee and back pains; 2. Sexual neurasthenia; 3. Dizziness and failing eyesight. Use 5-10 gm., as decoction. Root skins: 1. Fever of tuberculosis; 2. Coughs; 3. Haemoptysis, epistaxis. Use 10-15 gm., as decoction.

Prescriptions　　1. Failing eyesight: Lycium chinense fruits, 10 gm., steam with pork liver for consumption.

2. Weak "kidneys" and back pain: Lycium chinense fruits, Cibotium barometz rhizome 12 gm. each, as decoction.

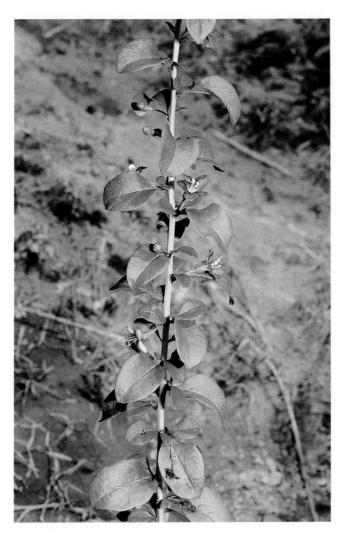

茄科、枸杞屬之灌木，高可達1米多。莖細長，柔弱，故常彎曲下垂，有棘刺。葉互生，或簇生於短枝上；葉片卵形、卵狀菱形或卵狀披針形，全緣。花常1至4朵簇生於葉腋；花萼鐘狀，3至5裂；花冠漏斗狀，筒部稍寬但短於檐部裂片，淡紫色，裂片有緣毛；雄蕊5枚，花絲基部密生絨毛。漿果卵狀或長橢圓狀卵形，長5至15毫米，紅色。種子腎形，黃色。花期：六月至十一月。

Solanaceae: Spiny shrubs, higher than 1m. Stems long and slender, hence often nodding. Leaves alternate, or appearing in clusters at branchlets; lamina ovate, ovate-rhombic or ovate-lanceolate; margin entire. Flowers axillary, often 1-4 in clusters; calyx campanulate, 3-5 lobed; corolla funnel-shaped, light purple, tube portion shorter than limb; stamens 5, filaments densely pubescent at base. Fruit a berry, red, oblong-ovoid, 5-15mm long, many-seeded. Seeds kidney-shaped, yellow. Flowering from June to November.

槍 刀 藥

Hypoestes purpurea (L.) Soland.

別　　名　刀槍藥。

生長環境　生於路邊灌木林中。

採集加工　藥用全株。全年可採，曬乾或鮮用。

性味功能　味微澀，性涼。清熱，止血。

主治用法　1. 支氣管炎，咳血；2. 外傷出血。每用 3 至 5 錢，水煎服。外用鮮品適量，搗爛敷患處。

Habitat　　　In roadside thickets.

Preparation　Use whole herb. Collect all year round. Dry under sun or use fresh.

Properties　　Slightly astringent tasting; cool. Anti-inflammatory, haemostatic.

Indications　1. Bronchitis, coughs; 2. Wound bleeding. Use 10-15 gm., as decoction. For external use, mash fresh herb as poultice.

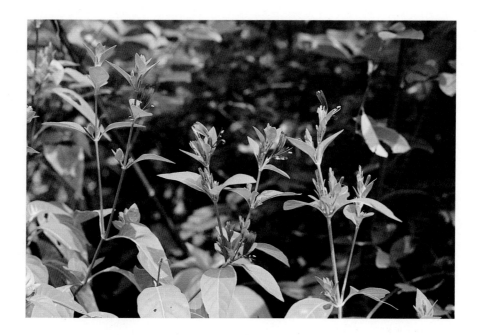

　　爵床科、槍刀藥屬之草本，高可達 1.5 米。葉對生，橢圓形至橢圓狀矩圓形；葉尖漸尖，葉基楔形；葉兩面均疏生短柔毛；葉緣具淺鈍齒。花序由1至5個聚傘花序集成，生於頂端或上方葉之葉腋；苞片倒披針狀矩圓形至倒卵狀矩圓形，有短柔毛，內有1至少數花朵；花萼裂片4，條狀披針形；花冠外生短柔毛。蒴果長約9毫米，上部有4顆種子。花期：三月。

　　Acanthaceae: Herbs, up to 1.5m high. Leaves opposite, elliptic or elliptical-oblong; apex acuminate, base cuneate; pilose on both surfaces; crenulate. 1-5 cymes in terminal inflorescence or axillary on upper stem; bracts oblanceolate-oblong to obovate-oblong, pilose, bracts surrounding 1 to a few flowers; sepals 4, linear lanceolate; corolla pilose outside. Capsules 9mm long, holding 4 seeds. Flowering in March.

松 葉 耳 草

Hedyotis pinifolia Wall.

別　　名　　了哥舌、鶇哥舌、鳥舌草、利尖草。

生長環境　　生於路旁、草地。

採集加工　　藥用全草。夏、秋採收，曬乾或鮮用。

性味功能　　味甘、淡，性平。清熱，消腫。

主治用法　　1. 跌打損傷；2. 癰瘡腫毒，蛇咬傷；3. 小兒疳積。每用 3 至 5 錢，水煎服。外用鮮品適量，搗敷患處。

主要成分　　全草含 β - 谷甾醇（β - sitosterol）、熊果酸（ursolic acid）等三萜類化合物。

Habitat　　On roadside and lawns.

Preparation　　Use whole herb. Collect in summer and autumn, dry under sun or use fresh.

Properties　　Sweet and bland tasting ; neutral. Anti-inflammatory, anti-swelling.

Indications　　1. Traumatic injury; 2. Boils and abscesses, snake bites; 3. Infantile malabsorption. Use 10-15 gm., as decoction. For external use, mash fresh herb as poultice.

Remarks　　The herb contains β-sitosterol, and ursolic acid.

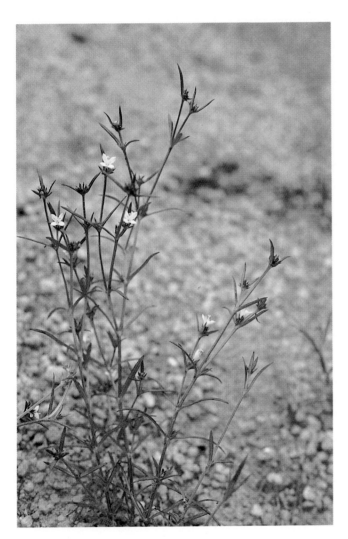

　　茜草科、耳草屬之一年生矮小披散草本。主莖頂生有多量銳四棱形之分枝。葉輪生，細條形，質硬挺直，兩面粗糙，只有中脈；托葉合生成鞘，頂端裂成數條刺毛。團傘花序，頂生或腋生，花 3 至 10 朵；花 4 數，苞片披針形；萼筒倒圓錐形，被毛，裂片鑽尖、具睫毛；花冠筒狀，裂片矩圓形；雄蕊生於花冠筒喉部。蒴果近卵形，被毛，熟時頂部開裂，有宿存之萼裂片。種子有棱。花期：五月至九月。

Rubiaceae: Annual spreading small herbs. Many 4-angled branchlets above the main stem. Leaves whorled, linear, firm, rough above and beneath, only midrib visible; stipules fused to form a sheath, apex splitting into several setae. Glomerules terminal or axillary, 3-10 flowered; flowers 4-merous, bracts lanceolate; calyx tubular, obconoid, hairy, lobes pointed, ciliate; corolla tubular, lobes oblong; stamens inserted to the corolla throat. Capsules subovoid, hairy, splitting at top when ripe; sepals persistent. Seeds ridged. Flowering from May to September.

蛇 根 草

Ophiorrhiza japonica Bl.

別　　名　日本蛇根草、四季花、血和散、雪裏梅。

生長環境　生於山谷林下陰濕地。

採集加工　藥用全草。全年可採，洗淨，曬乾或鮮用。

性味功能　味淡，性平。止咳祛痰，活血散瘀。

主治用法　1. 支氣管炎，肺結核咯血；2. 月經不調。每用5錢至1兩，水煎服。外用治扭挫傷。鮮品適量，搗爛外敷患處。

方　　例　1. 慢性支氣管炎：蛇根草8錢，水煎服。

2. 月經不調：蛇根草8錢，水煎服。

3. 扭挫傷：蛇根草1兩，水煎沖黃酒服；外用鮮草適量，加醋搗爛敷患處。

Habitat　　In moist and shaded land in valleys and under woods.

Preparation　　Use whole herb. Collect all year round, wash, dry under sun or use fresh.

Properties　　Bland tasting; neutral. Antitussive, expectorant; promotes circulation, resorbs bruises.

Indications　　1. Bronchitis, haemoptysis of pulmonary tuberculosis; 2. Irregular menstruation. Use 15-30 gm., as decoction. External use in sprains and strains. Mash sufficient amount of fresh herb as poultice.

Prescriptions　　1. Chronic bronchitis: Ophiorrhiza japonica 25 gm., as decoction.

2. Irregular menses: Ophiorrhiza japonica 25 gm., as decoction.

3. Strains and sprains: Ophiorrhiza japonica 30 gm., as decoction to be taken with wine. For external use, add vinegar to mashed fresh herb as poultice.

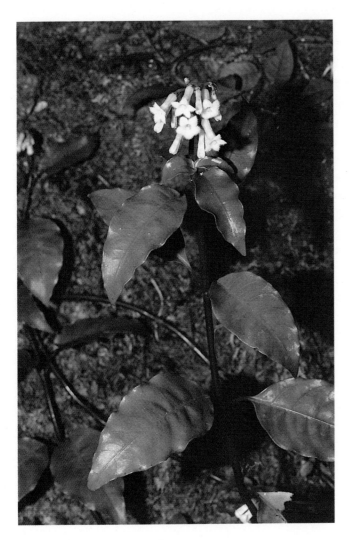

茜草科、蛇根草屬之直立草本。幼枝具棱，老枝則為圓柱形。葉對生，膜質，卵狀橢圓形，葉片無毛或上表面有疏短柔毛，側脈柔弱；葉柄纖細；托葉短小，早落。聚傘花序頂生，二歧分枝，花5至10朵，花5數；萼筒寬陀螺狀球形，裂片三角形，開展；花冠漏斗狀，裂片短尖，內面被微柔毛；雄蕊內藏。蒴果菱形，2裂，中部為萼筒圍繞。花期：三月至五月。

Rubiaceae: Erect herbs. Young stems ridged, old stems cylindrical. Leaves opposite, membranous, ovate-elliptic, lamina glabrous or sparsely pilose above, lateral veins delicate; petioles slender; stipules short and small, caducous. Cymes terminal, dichotomous, 5-10 flowered, flowers 5-merous; calyx tubular, broad turbinate-globose, lobes deltoid, open; corolla funnel-shaped, lobes mucronate, pilose inside; stamens wholly enclosed. Capsules rhombic, 2 valved, middle portion surrounded by calyx. Flowering from March to May.

珊 瑚 樹

Viburnum odoratissimum Ker-Gawl.

別　　名　　沙糖木、旱禾樹、香柄樹、楓飯樹、麻油香。

生長環境　　生於路邊灌木叢中。

採集加工　　藥用樹皮、根、葉。全年可採，曬乾或鮮用。

性味功能　　味辛，性溫。清熱，活絡。

主治用法　　1. 感冒；2. 風濕；3. 跌打腫痛，骨折。每用根3至5錢，水煎服。樹皮1至2兩，水煎服。葉外用治跌打損傷，鮮根適量，搗爛敷患處。

Habitat　　In roadside bushes.

Preparation　　Use bark, roots, leaves. Collect all year round, dry under sun or use fresh.

Properties　　Acrid tasting; warm. Promotes circulation.

Indications　　1. Common cold; 2. Rheumatism; 3. Traumatic injury, fractures. Use roots 10-15 gm., as decoction. Bark 30-60 gm., as decoction. Leaves useful for external treatment of traumatic injury. Fresh roots are mashed and used as poultice.

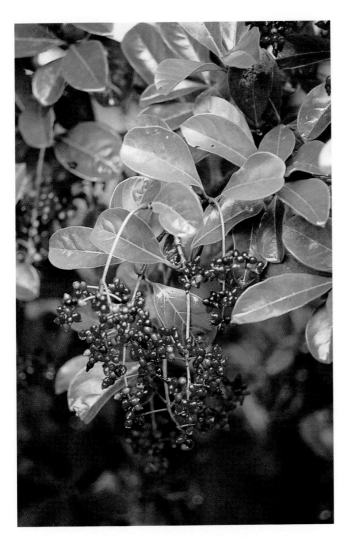

　　忍冬科、莢蒾屬之常綠灌木或
小喬木，高可達10米。葉革質，橢
圓形至橢圓狀矩圓形；葉緣為全緣
或具不規則淺波狀鈍齒；側脈4至5
對，在葉底面隆起。圓錐花序廣金
字塔形，腋生；花芳香；萼檐具5
淺鈍齒；花冠白色，輻狀，花冠筒
長約1毫米，裂片5，較花冠筒長2
至3倍；雄蕊5，着生於近花冠筒之
喉部。核果卵狀矩圓形，幼時紅，
成熟時黑。核有一深腹溝。花期：
四月。

Caprifoliaceae: Evergreen shrubs
or small trees, up to 10m high. Leaves
coriaceous, elliptic to elliptical-orbicular;
margin entire or irregularly crenulate;
lateral veins 4-5 pairs, elevated on the
lower surface. Flowers fragrant; panicles
axillary, pyramid shape; calyx crenulate,
5 toothed; corolla white, rotate, corolla
tube 1mm long, segments 5, 2-3 times
longer than the tube; stamens 5, inserted
to the throat. Drupe ovate-orbicular, red
when young, black at maturity. Seeds
with a deep abdominal groove.
Flowering in April.

杏香兔耳風
Ainsliaea fragrans Champ.

別　　名　一支香、兔耳風、兔耳一枝箭、金邊兔耳、朝天一柱香。

生長環境　生於山坡、林下陰濕處。

採集加工　藥用全草。全年可採，曬乾或鮮用。

性味功能　味苦，性寒。清熱解毒，利尿，止血，消積。

主治用法　1. 上呼吸道感染；2. 肺膿瘍，肺結核咯血；3. 小兒疳積，消化不良。每用5錢至1兩，水煎服。外用治瘡癤，乳腺炎，中耳炎，骨髓炎，毒蛇咬傷。鮮品搗爛外敷患處。

方　　例　1. 肺結核咯血：杏香兔耳風、魚腥草各 1 兩，功勞葉 5 錢，紅棗 5 枚，水煎服。

　　2. 小兒消化不良：杏香兔耳風3錢，白茅根1錢，水煎服，或研粉每次服1錢，每日服 3 次。

　　3. 急性骨髓炎：杏香兔耳風 2 兩，朱砂根、荔枝草各 1 兩，水煎服；渣外敷。

附　　註　本品水煎劑，對金黃色葡萄球菌有抑制作用。

Habitat　　On slopes, under woods in moist shaded area.

Preparation　　Use whole herb. Collect all year round, dry under sun or use fresh.

Properties　　Bitter tasting; cold. Anti-inflammatory, diuretic, haemostatic; promotes digestion.

Indications　　1. Upper respiratory tract infection; 2. Empyema, pulmonary tuberculosis with haemoptysis; 3. Infantile malabsorption, indigestion. Use 15-30 gm., as decoction. External use in furunculosis, mastitis, otitis media, osteomyelitis, poisonous snake bites. Mash fresh herb for topical application.

Prescriptions　　1. Pulmonary tuberculosis with haemoptysis: Ainsliaea fragrans, Houttuynia cordata, 30 gm. each, Ilex cornuta leaves 15 gm., red dates 5, as decoction.

2. Infantile indigestion: Ainsliaea fragrans 10 gm., Imperata cylindrica 3 gm., as decoction. May also grind into powder and take 3 gm. each time, 3 times daily.

Remarks　　This herb is bacteriostatic against Staphylococcus aureus.

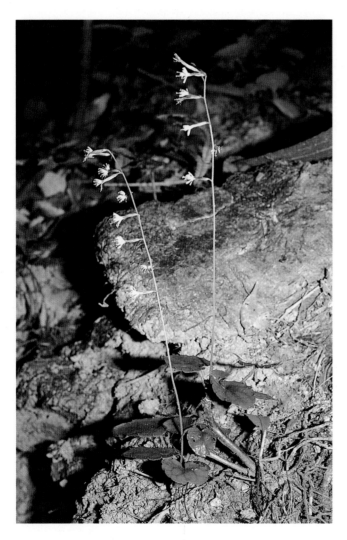

　　菊科、兔兒風屬之多年生草本。短根狀莖上具基生葉 5 至 10 塊，葉近輪生；葉片卵狀長橢圓形，先端圓鈍，葉基心臟形，全緣或略呈波狀，葉面綠色，葉背被棕色長絨毛或有時呈紫紅色；葉柄約與葉片等長，具棕色絨毛。頭狀花序細長，多數，排成總狀花叢，生於葉上方之直立莖上；總苞細筒狀；苞片多層；花呈筒狀，白色，略含杏仁氣味。瘦果栗褐色，具縱條紋及細毛。花期：四月。

Compositae: Perennial herbs. Basal leaves 5-10, in a sub-whorl, arising from a short rhizome; leaves oblong-elliptic, apex obtuse, base cordate, entire or slightly undulate; green above, brown villose or occasionally purplish red beneath; petiole nearly equalling lamina in length, brown villose. Flowers white, tubular, with a slight odour of almond, in racemes consisting of many slender capitula above the erect stem; involucre fine tubular, consisting of several layers. Fruit chestnut coloured, achene, with longitudinal ridges, pubescent. Flowering in April.

茵　陳

Artemisia scoparia Waldst. et Kit.

別　　名　黃蒿、濱蒿、豬毛蒿、北茵陳、綿茵陳。

生長環境　生於海邊沙地。

採集加工　藥用幼苗。春季幼苗 6 至 7 厘米高時採集，去根，曬乾。

性味功能　味苦、辛，性微寒。清熱，利尿，退黃疸。

主治用法　1. 黃疸型肝炎；2. 膽囊炎；3. 蕁麻疹，藥疹，濕疹。每用 3 錢至 1 兩，水煎服。外用適量煎水洗患處。

方　　例　1. 黃疸型肝炎，大便秘結：茵陳 1 兩，山梔子、生大黃、車前草、板藍根各 3 錢，水煎服。

2. 蕁麻疹，藥疹：茵陳、土茯苓、綠豆各 1 兩，紅棗 10 枚，水煎服。

3. 膽囊炎急性發作：茵陳、蒲公英各 1 兩，黃芩，山梔子、生大黃、枳殼、澤瀉、鬱金各 3 錢，水煎服，另加玄明粉 2 錢沖服。

主要成分　含揮發油，油中主要成分為側柏醇、丁醛、糖醛、α - 蒎烯等。

Habitat　　　　On sandy beaches.

Preparation　　Use young shoots. Collect in spring when young shoots are 6-7 cm high. Remove roots and dry under sun.

Properties　　　Bitter and acrid tasing; mildly cold. Anti-inflammatory, duretic; relieves jaundice.

Indications　　1. Icteric hepatitis; 2. Cholecystitis; 3. Urticaria, eczema, drug eruption. Use 10-30 gm., as decoction. For external usse, boil in water for washing.

Prescriptions　1. Icteric hepatitis, constipation: Artemisia scoparia, Gardenia jasminoides fruits, Rheum officinale, Plantago major, Isatis tinctoria roots, 10 gm. each, as decoction.

2. Urticaria, drug eruption: Artemisia scoparia, Smilax glabra, Phaseolus radiatus seeds, 30 gm. each, red dates 10, as decoction.

3. Acute eholecystitis: Artemisia scoparia, Taraxacum mongolicum, 30 gm. each, Gardenia jasminoides fruits, Rheum officinale, Citrus aurantium rind, Alisma orientalis, Curcuma aromatica, 10 gm. each, Natrii Sulfas Exsiccatus 6 gm., as decoction.

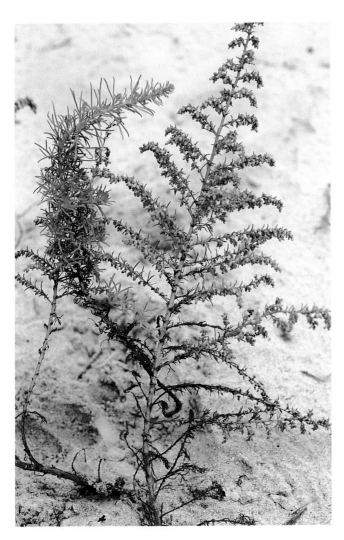

　　菊科、蒿屬之一或二年生草本，高約 90 厘米。莖直立，頗多斜升之分枝，被微柔毛或近無毛；不育枝密集，且葉較大塊。葉密集；莖上部之葉 3 裂或不裂；中部之葉 1 或 2 次羽狀全裂，且裂片極細；下部之葉與不育枝之葉同形狀，葉片短圓形，2 或 3 次羽狀全裂，裂片狹長。頭狀花序極多數，在莖及側枝上排列成複總狀花序；外層有 5 至 7 朵雌性能育花，內層有 4 朵不育花。瘦果。花期：六月。

Compositae: Annual or biennial herbs, up to 90cm high. Stems erect, oblique branchlets numerous, pilose or subglabrous; sterile branchlets dense, leaves larger. Leaves dense; upper leaves trifid or entire; middle leaves pinnate or bipinnate, pinnae small; leaves on lower stem similar in shape to those on sterile branches, suborbicular, bipinnate or tripinnate, pinnae linear. Numerous capitula forming a compound raceme on the stem as well as on the branches; 5-7 fertile pistillates on the outside layer, 4 sterile flowers inside. Fruits achenes. Flowering in June.

大頭艾納香

Blumea megacephala (Rand.) Chang et Tseng

別　　名　白花九里明、華艾納香、東風草、黃花地膽草。

生長環境　生於山坡灌木叢中。

採集加工　藥用全草。全年可採，曬乾或鮮用。

性味功能　味微苦、淡，性微溫。祛風除濕，活血調經。

主治用法　1. 風濕骨痛，跌打腫痛；2. 產後血崩，月經不調。每用5錢至1兩，水煎服。外用治瘡癤，鮮品適量，搗敷患處。

主要成分　含黃酮類。

Habitat　　On slopes and mong thickets.

Preparation　　Use whole herb. Collect all year round, dry under sun or use fresh.

Properties　　Slightly bitter and bland tasting; mildly warm. Antirheumatic; promotes circulation, regulates menses.

Indications　　1. Rheumatic bone pains, traumatic injury; 2. Postpartum haemorrhage, irregular menses. Use 15-30 gm., as decoction. For external use in boils and pyodermas, apply mashed fresh herb to lesion.

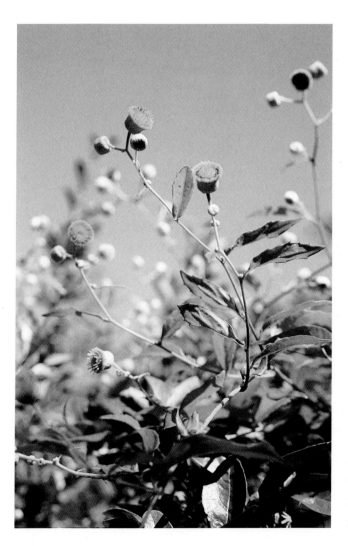

菊科、艾納香屬之攀援狀草質藤本或基部木質。莖多分枝，具明顯溝紋，被疏毛或後脫毛。葉互生；莖上部之葉較細小，葉柄極短，莖下部及中部之葉柄較長，葉片卵形，卵狀長圓形或長橢圓形；葉緣具疏細齒或點狀齒；葉面被疏毛或後脫毛，有光澤；網脈極明顯。頭狀花序疏散；通常1至7個腋生，排成總狀或近傘房狀花序，再排成大型具葉之圓錐花序；花黃色。瘦果具10棱。花期：八月至十二月。

Compositae: Climbing herbs or woody at base. Stem many-branched, with distinct furrows, covered sparsely with hairs which are later shed. Leaves alternate; leaves at upper stem small, petioles short; leaves at mid- and lower stem with longer petioles; lamina ovate, ovate-oblong or oblong elliptic; margin serrulate or crenulate; lamina covered sparsely with hairs which are later shed, glossy; reticulate venation distinct. Flowers yellow, in 1-7 axillary heads forming racemous or sub-corymbose inflorescences which in turn form a large leafy panicle. Achenes with 10 ridges. Flowering from August to December.

金 盞 菊

Calendula officinalis L.

別　　名　金盞花、山金菊、燈盞花。

生長環境　栽培於庭園中。

採集加工　藥用根、花。夏季採花，秋季採根，曬乾或鮮用。

性味功能　味淡，性平。根：活血散瘀，止痛。花：涼血止血。

主治用法　根：癥瘕，疝氣，胃寒疼痛。花：腸風便血，目赤腫痛。每用根1至2兩，花5至10朵，水煎服。

方　　例　1. 胃寒疼痛：金盞菊鮮根2兩，水煎服。

2. 腸風便血：金盞菊鮮花10朵，冰糖少許，水煎服。

主要成分　花含金盞黃素（flavochrome）、胡蘿蔔素、番茄烴等。根含三萜烯貳類化合物金盞花貳B，對大鼠關節炎，有明顯的抗炎和抗潰瘍作用。

附　　註　歐洲民間把本品外用於皮膚黏膜各種炎症。內服治潰瘍病，胃炎，肝膽疾患；用於消化道腫瘤可減輕症狀，改善食慾，睡眠；亦有用於月經不調。

Habitat　　Cultivated in gardens.

Preparation　　Use roots and flowers. Collect flowers in summer, roots in autumn, dry under sun or use fresh.

Properties　　Bland tasting, neutral. Roots promote circulation and resorb bruises; analgesic. Flowers are heamostatic.

Indications　　Roots: Scars, hernias, epigastric pain. Flowers: Sore eyes. Use roots 30-60 gm., flowers 5-10, as decoction.

Prescriptions　1. Epigastric pain: Calendula officinalis fresh roots 60 gm., as decoction.

2. Bleeding haemorrhoids: Calendula officinalis fresh flowers 10 pieces, add small amount of rock sugar, as decoction.

Remarks　　This herb is popularly used in European countryside as treatment for inflammation of skin and mucous membrane. Internal use in ulcers, gastritis, liver and gall bladder ailments. Useful in alleviating symptoms in tumours of the gastrointestinal tract; in improving appetite and enhancing the state of sleep. Also effective in regulating menses.

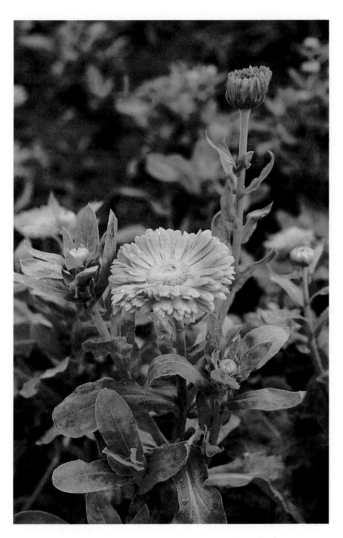

　　菊科、金盞花屬之一年生或二年生草本，高約40厘米。全株被短毛。莖上有縱棱。葉互生，長倒卵形，淡綠色，葉質柔軟，無葉柄。頭狀花序，單個頂生於主莖及分枝上，直徑7厘米；花異性，放射狀；緣花黃色或橙色，舌狀，1至2列；盤花不結實；總苞闊大，苞片1至2列。瘦果禿淨。花期：七月。

Compositae: Annual or biennial herbs, about 40cm high, whole plant pubescent. Stems with longitudinal ridges. Leaves alternate, oblong-obovate, light green, soft, sessile. Capitulum solitary, terminal on main stem and branches, 7cm in diameter; flowers of two types, radial; ray flowers yellow or orange, ligulate, in 1 or 2 rows; disk flowers sterile; involucre large, bracts in 1 or 2 rows. Achenes glabrous. Flowering in July.

茼　蒿

Chrysanthemum segetum L.

別　　名　同蒿、同蒿菜、南茼蒿、蓬蒿菜。

生長環境　多為栽培。

採集加工　藥用嫩莖葉。冬、春採收，鮮用。

性味功能　味甘，性平。和脾胃，利二便，消痰飲。

主治用法　1. 熱咳；2. 消化不良，便秘；3. 小便不利。每用鮮品 1 至 2 兩，水煎服。泄瀉者忌用。

方　　例　熱咳：鮮茼蒿3兩，水煎去渣，加冰糖適量，溶化後，分2次飲用。

主要成分　莖和葉含多種氨基酸：絲氨酸、天門冬素、蘇氨酸、丙氨酸、谷氨酰胺、纈氨酸、亮氨酸、脯氨酸、天冬氨酸、谷氨酸、β-丁氨酸、苯丙氨酸等。

附　　註　茼蒿一般作蔬菜食。

Habitat　　Mostly cultivated.

Preparation　　Use the tender leaves and stem. Collect in winter and spring, use fresh.

Properties　　Sweet tasting; neutral. Soothing to the stomach and spleen; promotes bowel and urine excretion, reduces sputum.

Indications　　1. Dry coughs; 2. Indigestion, constipation; 3. Oliguria. Use fresh herb 30-60 gm. as decoction. Contraindicated in those with chronic diarrhea.

Prescription　　Dry coughs: Chrysanthemum segetum 100 gm., as decoction, discard the residue, add rock sugar, and divide into 2 doses.

Remarks　　This is usually used as vegetable.

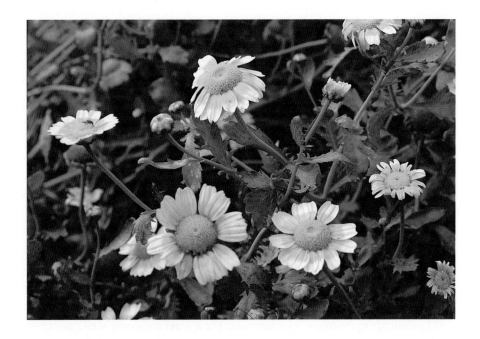

　　菊科、茼蒿屬直立草本，高20至60厘米。植株光滑無毛或幾無毛，莖直立，富肉質。葉橢圓形，倒卵狀披針形或倒卵狀橢圓形；葉面深綠色；葉稍呈肉質；葉緣具不規則之大鋸齒，偶有成羽狀淺裂者；葉基楔形，無葉柄。頭狀花序頂生，花序柄長5厘米，花黃色。內層總苞片膜質擴大幾成附片狀；舌片長1.5厘米；舌狀花瘦果有2條具狹翅的側肋，間肋不明顯，每面3至6條；管狀花瘦果有肋約10條。花期：十一月。

　　Compositae: Erect herbs, glabrous or subglabrous, 20-60cm high. Stem erect, fleshy. Leaves elliptic, obovate-lanceolate or obovate-elliptic; dark-green above; subcarnose; margin irregularly serrate, occasionally shallowly pinnate; base cuneiform, sessile. Flowers yellow; heads terminal, peduncle 5cm long; inner involucre membranous, enlarged as appendages; ligule 1.5cm long; achenes of ray flowers with 2 narrow-winged ridges with again 3-6 inconspicuous ridges between them; achenes of tubular flowers with 10 ridges. Flowering in November.

大 麗 花

Dahlia pinnata Cav.

別　　名　大麗菊、大理菊、洋芍藥、芍藥、西番蓮、天竺牡丹。
生長環境　多栽培於庭園。
採集加工　藥用塊根。夏、秋採，曬乾或鮮用。
性味功能　味甘，性平。消炎。
主治用法　1. 瘡瘍腫毒；2. 跌打腫痛。外用鮮品搗敷患處。
主要成分　根含菊糖，醫藥上與葡萄糖功效相同。
附　　註　香港常把本品稱為芍藥，但與中藥常用毛茛科的芍藥（Paeonia
lactiflora）（有止痛，養血，調經功效），完全不同，功效大異，切勿誤用。

Habitat　　Mostly cultivated in gardens.
Preparation　Use tubers. Collect in summer and autumn, dry under sun or use fresh.
Properties　Sweet tasting; neutral. Anti-inflammatory.
Indications　1. Pyodermas; 2. Traumatic injury. Mash fresh herb for external use.
Remarks　In Hong Kong, this herb is often mistaken as Paeonia lactiflora as the Chinese name of the latter（芍藥）and one of the Chinese names of this herb（洋芍藥）are very close. However, they belong to different families and also have very different medicinal properties (Paeonia lactiflora belongs to the family Ranunculaceae and has the properties of analgesia, tonic, and regulating the menses). Care should be taken not to mix up the two in their applications.

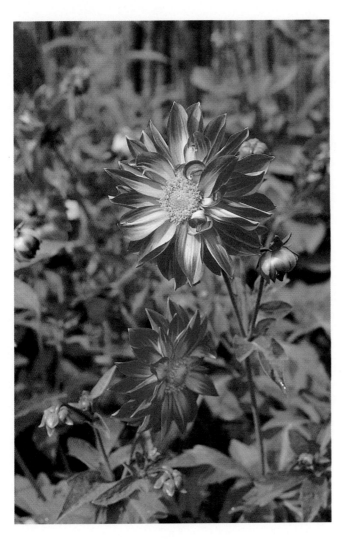

菊科、大麗花屬之多年生草本，塊根棒狀且巨大。莖直立，粗壯，多分枝。葉互生，1至3回羽狀全裂，莖上部之葉有時不分裂，裂片卵形或長圓狀卵形，葉背面灰綠色。花序梗長，頭狀花序大型且重，故常下垂；花序外圍有無性或雌性小花，花舌狀，常卵形，頂端有不明顯之3齒；花有白色，紅色或紫色；花序中央之兩性花多數，花管狀，黃色，頂端有5齒。瘦果長圓形，黑色。花期：六月至十二月。

Compositae: Perennial herbs, root-tuber clavate, large. Stems erect, shout, branchy. Leaves alternate; pinnate, bipinnate or tripinnate, upper leaves occasionally simple, pinnae ovate or oblong-ovate, greyish green beneath. Rachis of inflorescence long, capitulum large and heavy, hence usually nodding; ray florets asexual or pistillate, ligulate, white, red or violet, tip inconspicuously 3-toothed; central flowers bisexual, numerous, tubular, yellow, tip 5-toothed. Achenes oblong, black. Flowering from June to December.

山 萵 苣

Lactuca indica L.

別　　名　土萵苣、苦菜、苦芥菜、野生菜、敗醬草。

生長環境　生於向陽之路邊、荒野。

採集加工　藥用全草或根。夏、秋採集，曬乾或鮮用。

性味功能　味苦，性寒。有小毒。清熱解毒。

主治用法　1. 扁桃體炎；2. 乳腺炎，子宮頸炎，瘡癤；3. 痔瘡下血。每用3至5錢，水煎服。外用適量。

方　　例　1. 扁桃體炎：山萵苣全草1兩，水煎，分2次服。

2. 乳癰，瘡癤：鮮山萵苣全草適量，搗爛外敷患處。

主要成分　全草含β-香樹脂酮醇（β-amyrenyl）、吉曼尼醇（germanicyl）、乙酸蒲公英醇酯等。根含山萵苣素（lactucin）、莨菪鹼等。

附　　註　山萵苣可供食用，取幼苗及嫩莖葉，用沸水快速燙熟，撈起切絲，拌以各種調味料食用。

Habitat　　　On sunny roadside and in the wild.

Preparation　Use roots or whole herb. Collect all year round, dry under sun or use fresh.

Properties　　Bitter tasting; cold. Slightly toxic, anti-inflammatory.

Indications　1. Tonsillitis; 2. Mastitis, cervicitis, furunculosis; 3. Hammerhead with bleeding. Use 10-15 gm., as decoction. Use suitable amount for external application.

Prescriptions　1. Tonsillitis: Lactuca indica whole herb 30 gm., as decoction, divide into two doses.

2. Breast abscess, furunculosis: Mash sufficient fresh herb and use as poultice.

Remarks　　Lactuca indica is also used as food, The young shoots and tender leaves are scalded in hot water, then sliced into fine segments and mixed with seasoning.

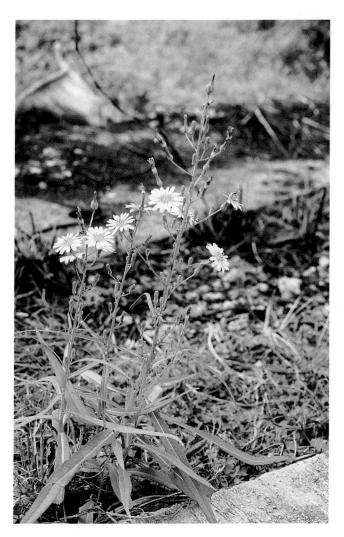

菊科、萵苣屬之二年生草本，高約 120 厘米。主莖上部有分枝。葉密集，無柄，具狹窄膜片狀長毛；葉形多變化：條形、長橢圓狀條形、條狀披針形等；羽狀或倒向羽狀之全裂或深裂，裂片邊緣缺刻狀或鋸齒狀針刺；葉基戟形半抱莖；莖下部葉於花期枯萎。頭狀花序有小花 25 朵，於莖枝頂排成寬或窄之圓錐花序；舌狀花淡黃或白色。瘦果黑色，扁，內彎，喙短，冠毛白色。花期：二月。

Compositae: Biennial herbs, about 120cm high, upper part of the stem branchy. Leaves dense, sessile, possessing long narrow membranous hairs; shape various; linear, oblong-elliptic linear or linear lanceolate; pinnate or reverse pinnate, lobed or deeply lobed, margin incised or bristly-toothed; base hastate, subamplexicaul; lower leaves wilt at bloom. Capitula of 25 florets arranged in terminal panicles; ray florets light yellow or white. Achenes black, compressed, recurved inwards, beak short, pappus white. Flowering in February.

大 頭 橐 吾

Ligularia japonica (Thunb.) Less.

別　　名　　兔打傘、猴巴掌、望江南。

生長環境　　生於山坡、林緣陰濕處。

採集加工　　藥用根或全草。夏季採集，曬乾或鮮用。

性味功能　　味辛，性微溫。活血，解毒，消腫。

主治用法　　1. 跌打損傷；2. 瘡癤腫毒；3. 毒蛇咬傷。每用根 5 錢至 1 兩，水煎服。外用適量。

方　　例　　1. 跌打損傷：大頭橐吾根 1 兩，酒、水各半煎服；同時取鮮草適量加白酒搗爛外敷。

2. 瘡瘍腫毒：大頭橐吾根適量，白糖少許，共搗爛外敷，早晚各換藥一次。

主要成分　　全株含呋喃倍半萜（furanosesquiterpenes）。

Habitat　　On damp shady soil of slopes and woods.

Preparation　　Use roots or whole herb. Collect in summer, dry under sun or use fresh.

Properties　　Acrid tasting; slightly warm. Promotes circulation; anti-inflammatory; reduces swelling.

Indications　　1. Traumatic injury; 2. Boils and furuncles; 3. Poisonous snake bites. Use roots 15-30 gm., as decotion. Use suitable amount externally.

Prescriptions　　1.Traumatic injury: Ligularia japonica roots 30 gm., brew in equal amounts of wine and water. Also mash suitable amount of fresh leaves to blend with white wine and use as poultice.

2. Boils and pyodermas: Ligularia japonica roots mixed with white sugar for topical use twice daily.

Remarks　　The whole herb contains furanosesquiterpenes.

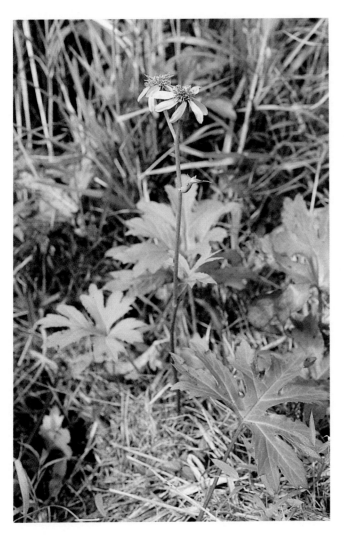

　　菊科、橐吾屬之多年生直立草本，高可達 1 米。莖無毛或具蜘蛛絲狀毛。植株上方之葉片小，掌狀深裂，短葉柄抱莖；植株下方之葉片大，掌狀深裂，裂片再掌狀淺裂，葉緣具小鋸齒，葉柄長達 70 厘米而基部擴大抱莖。花序傘房狀，總花梗長，被密短捲毛；頭狀花序 2 至 8 個，直徑達 10 厘米；總苞寬鐘狀，被密短毛；舌狀花黃色，1 層，約 10 朵；筒狀花多數。瘦果，冠毛紅褐色。花期：十一月。

Compositae: Perennial erect herbs, up to 1m high. Stems glabrous or arachnoid-pilose. Upper leaves small, palmately deep-lobed, petioles short amplexicaul; lower leaves large, palmately deep-lobed, each lobe again palmately shallow-incised, margin serrulate, petiole up to 70cm long and enlarged at base, amplexicaul. Umbels on long peduncles which are covered with short lanate hairs; heads 2 to 8, 10cm in diameter; involucre broadly campanulate, densely pubescent; ray florets about 10, yellow, in 1 whorl; disc florets numerous. Achenes with reddish brown pappus. Flowering in November.

風　毛　菊

Saussurea japonica (Thunb.) DC.

別　　名　　八面風、八楞木、八棱麻、青竹標。

生長環境　　生於山坡、丘陵草叢中。

採集加工　　藥用全草。夏、秋季採收，曬乾用。

性味功能　　味苦、辛，性寒。祛風濕，清熱，活血。

主治用法　　1. 風濕關節炎，腰腿痛；2. 跌打損傷；3. 肺熱咳嗽。每用 5 錢至 1 兩，水煎服。外用適量，煎水洗患處。

方　　例　　1. 風濕關節炎：風毛菊、忍冬藤、桑枝各 5 錢，水煎服。

2. 跌打損傷：風毛菊 1 兩，徐長卿 5 錢，泡酒服。

Habitat　　On slopes, hills, and among bushes.

Preparation　　Use whole herb. Collect in summer and autumn, dry under sun.

Properties　　Bitter and acrid tasting; cold. Anti-rheumatic, anti-inflammatory, promotes circulation.

Indications　　1. Rheumatic arthralgia, low back pain; 2. Traumatic injury; 3. Coughs. Use 15-30 gm., as decoction. For external use, boil suitable quantity of herb in water for washing.

Prescriptions　　1. Rheumatic arthralgia: Saussurea japonica, Lonicera japonica vines, Morus alba branches, 15 gm. each , as decoction.

2. Traumatic injury: Saussurea japonica 30 gm., Cynanchum paniculatum 15 gm., brew in wine for oral consumption.

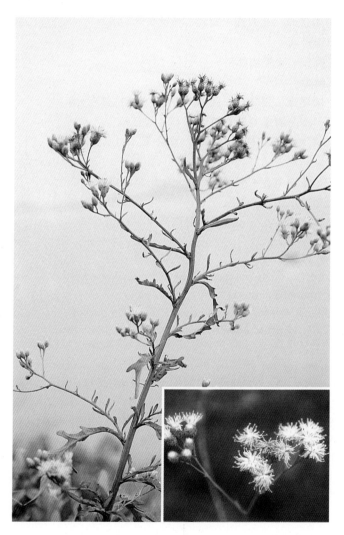

　　菊科、風毛菊屬之二年生草本，高可達150厘米。根紡錘狀。莖直立，粗壯，上部具分枝，被短微毛及腺點。基生葉及下部葉有長柄，矩圓形或橢圓形，羽狀分裂，中裂片矩圓狀披針形，側裂片狹矩圓形，葉兩面有短微毛和腺點；莖上部之葉漸小，橢圓形、披針形或條狀披針形，羽狀分裂或全緣。頭狀花序多數，排成密傘房狀，小花紫色。瘦果之冠毛淡褐色，外層糙毛狀，內層羽毛狀。花期：八月至十一月。

Compositae: Biennial herbs, up to 150cm high. Roots spindle-like. Stems erect, stout, upper part branchy, pubescent, punctate. Basal leaves and lower leaves long petioled, oblong or elliptic, pinnate, middle pinna short round lanceolate, lateral pinnae narrow oblong, pubescent and punctate on both surfaces; upper leaves gradually smaller, elliptic, lanceolate or linear-lanceolate, entire or pinnate. Capitula, numerous, in corymbose formation, florets purple. Achenes with light brown pappus, outer layer hispid, inner layer feathery. Flowering from August to November.

苣 蕒 菜

Sonchus arvensis L.

別　　名　山苦蕒、野苦蕒、牛舌頭、北敗醬、裂葉苦蕒菜。

生長環境　生於山坡、村旁和田野間。

採集加工　藥用全草。春、夏採收，曬乾或鮮用。

性味功能　味苦，性寒。清熱解毒。

主治用法　1. 急性咽喉炎；2. 闌尾炎，腸炎；3. 菌痢，痔瘡。每用5錢至1兩，水煎服。外用治瘡癤腫毒，乳腺炎。鮮品適量搗爛外敷患處。

方　　例　1. 細菌性痢疾：苣蕒菜、馬齒莧、刺莧菜、狗肝菜，均用鮮品各 1 兩，水煎，分兩次服。

2. 瘡癤腫毒，乳腺炎：苣蕒菜、犁頭草各 1 兩，水煎服。外用鮮品搗敷。

3. 痔瘡發炎：苣蕒菜鮮品 4 兩，煎水薰洗患處。

主要成分　全草含 α - 和 β - 山萵苣醇（lactucerol）、甘露醇（mannitol）等。

Habitat　　On slopes, village edges and fields.

Preparation　　Use whole herb. Collect in spring and summer, dry under sun or use fresh.

Properties　　Bitter tasting, cold. Anti-inflammatory.

Indications　　1. Acute pharyngitis; 2. Appendicitis, enteritis; 3. Bacillary dysentery, haemorrhoids. Use 15-30 gm., as decoction. External use in furunculosis, mastitis. Mash fresh herbs for local application.

Prescriptions　1. Bacillary dysentery: Sonchus arvensis, Portulaca oleracea, Amaranthus spinosus, Dicliptera chinensis, all in the fresh state, 30 gm. each, as decoction, divide into two doses.

2. Furunculosis, mastitis: Sonchus arvensis, Viola inconspicua, 30 gm. each, as decoction. Mash fresh herbs for external application.

3. Haemorrhoids inflammation: Fresh Sonchus arvensis 120 gm., boil in water to wash affected parts.

Remarks　　This herb contains alpha and beta lactucerol and mannitol.

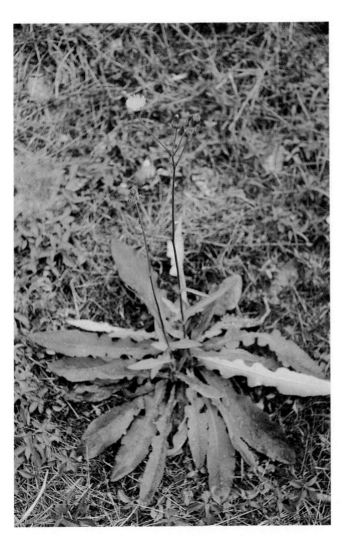

菊科、苦苣菜屬之多年生草本，具乳汁。具匍匐莖及地上莖；後者直立，高 30 至 80 厘米。葉互生；長圓狀披針形；葉緣具稀疏缺刻或三角狀淺裂。匍匐莖上葉之葉基漸狹成柄；莖生葉無柄，葉基成耳廓狀抱莖。花黃色，頭狀花序頂生，花序梗及總苞片均具腺毛；總苞鐘狀，苞片數層，最內層苞片薄、具膜質緣，披針形；花呈舌狀；雄蕊 5，花藥基部相連；子房下位。瘦果長橢圓形。花期：八月。

Compositae: Perennial herbs, lactiferous, with stolons as well as erect stems, the latter 30-80cm high. Leaves alternate; oblong-lanceolate; margins remotely incised or shallowly deltoid-lobed. Petioles of leaves on stolons attenuate; leaves on erect stem sessile, possessing auricular bases which clasp the stem. Flowers yellow, ligule, in terminal capitula, rachis and involucre with glandular hairs; involucre campanulate, bracts in several whorls; inner whorl thin, margin membranous, lanceolate; stamens 5, anthers connate at base; ovary inferior. Achene long ellipsoidal. Flowering in August.

天 文 草

Spilanthes acmella (L.) Murr.

別　　名　金鈕扣、山天文草、散血草、雨傘草、擬千日菊。

生長環境　生於田野濕地、水溝邊、路旁。

採集加工　藥用全草。全年可採，鮮用或曬乾備用。

性味功能　味辛，性溫。有麻舌感。止咳，定喘，解毒，止痛。

主治用法　1. 感冒咳嗽，慢性支氣管炎；2. 哮喘，百日咳；3. 瘧疾，牙痛；4. 腸炎，痢疾。每用3至5錢，水煎服或研末，每服2至3分。孕婦慎用。外用治癰癤腫毒，跌打損傷，毒蛇咬傷，狗咬傷。鮮品適量搗爛外敷患處。

方　　例　慢性支氣管炎：天文草3錢，木蝴蝶1錢，水煎分兩次服。

主要成分　全草含 α- 和 β- 香樹脂醇、蜂花醇（myricyl alcohol）、豆甾醇、谷甾醇 -o-β-D- 葡萄糖甙。

附　　註　本品可製成50%注射液，用於局部浸潤麻醉。個別患者注射後，會出現全身皮膚過敏現象，可用一般抗過敏藥治療。

Habitat　　In fields, along gullies and roadside.

Preparation　　Use whole herb. Collect all year round, use fresh or dry under sun for storage.

Properties　　Acrid tasting; warm. Astringent feeling to the tongue. Antitussive, anti-asthmatic, anti-inflammatory, analgesic.

Indications　　1. Colds and coughs, chronic bronchitis; 2. Asthma, pertussis; 3. Malaria, toothache; 4. Enteritis, dysentery. Use 10-15 gm., as decoction, or pulverize and take 0.5-1 gm. Contraindicated in pregnancy. External use in boils and pyodermas, traumatic injury, snake bites, dog bites. Crush fresh herb for topical use.

Prescription　　Chronic bronchitis: Spilanthes acmella 10 gm., Oroxylum indicum seeds 3 gm., as decoction to be taken in 2 doses.

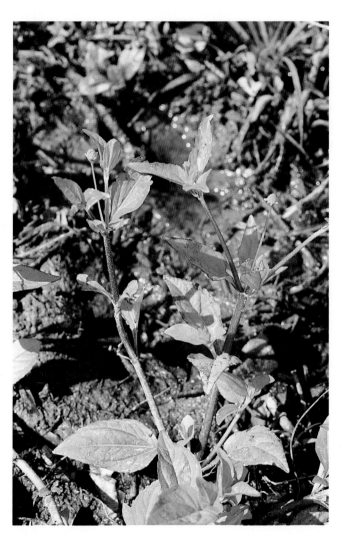

　　菊科、金鈕扣屬之一年生草本。主莖直立，分枝斜升，略被毛。葉對生，卵形至卵狀披針形，主脈 3 條，葉緣具鈍鋸齒或近全緣。頭狀花序卵形，1 至 3 個頂生，總花梗細長；總苞片 2 層，卵狀披針形；花托圓柱形或卵形；托片具短柄，包圍小花；花異形，黃色。瘦果倒卵形，頂端微凹，背部扁平，腹部稍隆起，表面被瘤狀疏毛，邊緣具向上的睫毛；冠毛芒狀。花期：四月至十一月。

Compositae: Annual herbs. Main stem erect, branches oblique, nearly glabrous. Leaves opposite, ovate to ovate-lanceolate, mid-ribs 3, margin with blunt teeth or subentire. Flowers yellow, ovate heads 1-3, terminal, peduncle long and slender; bracts of involucre 2 whorled, ovate-lanceolate; receptacle cylindrical or ovoid, bracts short-stalked, surrounding the florets. Achene obovoid, apex retuse, enlarged at the middle, surface covered sparsely with tuberculate hairs, margins with upward-pointing ciliate hairs; pappus spike-like. Flowering from April to November.

趾 葉 栝 樓

Trichosanthes pedata Merr. et Chun

別　　名	叉指葉栝蔞、石蟾蜍、瓜蔞、趾葉栝蔞。
生長環境	生於山谷疏林和路邊灌木叢中。
採集加工	藥用塊根或全草。秋季採挖，切段，曬乾。
性味功能	味甘、苦，性涼。清熱解毒。
主治用法	1. 咽喉腫痛；2. 癰瘡癤腫；3. 蛇咬傷。每用 3 至 5 錢，水煎服。
主要成分	種子含油 56.2% 和脂肪酸等。
附　　註	雲南民間用果實代栝蔞（T. uniflora）入藥。本品為香港新記錄植物。

Habitat	In sparse woods of ravines and roadside thickets.
Preparation	Use tuber or whole herb. Collect in autumn, cut into segment, dry under sun.
Properties	Sweet and bitter tasting; cool. Anti-inflammatory.
Indications	1. Sore throat; 2. Furuncles and carbuncles; 3. Snake bites. Use 10-15 gm., as decoction.
Remarks	This is a newly recorded species in Hong Kong.

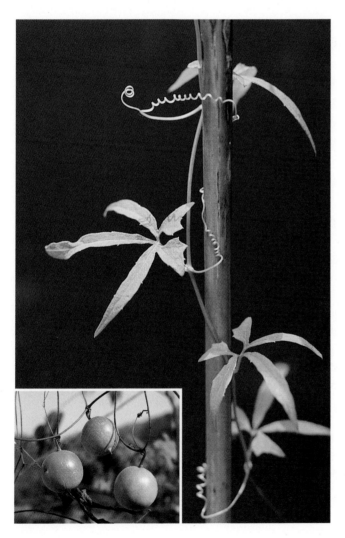

　　葫蘆科、栝樓屬之攀援藤本，
莖草質。捲鬚常分 2 叉；葉為鳥足
狀，小葉 5 片，中間小葉卵狀披針
形，兩側小葉近菱形或兩側不對稱
之側狹卵形，葉面及葉背均佈有顆
粒狀小凸點。雌雄異株；雄花生於
總狀花序上；苞片倒卵形或菱狀卵
形，銳裂；花萼裂片矩圓形，漸
尖，緣有小齒或近全緣；花瓣流蘇
狀；雄蕊 3。果球形，直徑約 5 厘
米，表面平滑。種子卵形或倒卵
形，稍脹大。花期：六月至八月。

Cucurbitaceae: Climbers, stems
herbal, tendrils often 2-branched. Leaves
unguiculate, leaflets 5, the middle one
ovate-lanceolate, the lateral ones
subrhomboid or asymmetrically
narrowly ovate, tuberculate above and
beneath. Dioecious; staminates in
raceme, bracts obovate or rhombic ovate,
acutely-lobed; sepal lobes oblong-
orbicular, acuminate, margins with fine
teeth or subentire; petals fimbriate;
stamens 3. Fruits globose, 5cm across,
glabrous. Seeds ovoid or obovoid,
slightly swollen. Flowering from June to
August.

蘆　根

Phragmites communis (L.) Trin.

別　　名　　水蓢蒩、水蘆荻、蘆葦根、葦子草、葦根、蒹葭。

生長環境　　生於河岸或沼澤中。

採集加工　　藥用根狀莖。夏、秋採挖，去地上莖，切段，曬乾或鮮用。

性味功能　　味甘，性寒。清熱解毒，生津，利尿。

主治用法　　1. 感冒、流感高熱，胃熱嘔吐；2. 氣管炎，肺炎，肺膿瘍；3. 鼻出血，牙齦出血；4. 尿路感染；5. 酒、魚蟹、河豚中毒。每用 5 錢至 1 兩，水煎服。

方　　例　　1. 肺膿瘍：鮮蘆根 2 兩，魚腥草 1 兩，冬瓜仁 8 錢，苡仁 5 錢，桃仁 2 錢，水煎服。

2. 熱病發熱傷津，口乾，舌燥，煩渴：「五汁飲」：蘆根、梨、荸薺、藕、麥冬（或蔗），均用鮮品適量搗汁，和勻涼服，或燉溫服。

主要成分　　含薏苡素、5% 蛋白質、1% 脂肪、51% 碳水化合物等。

Habitat　　On river banks and in swamps.

Preparation　　Use rhizomes. Collect in summer and autumn, discard the stems that grow above ground level, cut into segments, dry under sun or use fresh.

Properties　　Sweet tasting; cold. Anti-inflammatory; increases salivary secretion, diuretic.

Indications　　1. Influenza, high fever of epidemic influenza, vomiting; 2. Bronchitis, pneumonitis, empyema; 3. Epistaxis, gum bleeding; 4. Urinary tract infection; 5. Poisoning by alcohol, seafood, crabs, and "puffer fish". Use 15-30 gm., as decoction.

Prescriptions　　1. Empyema: Fresh Phragmites communis roots 60 gm., Houttuynia cordata 30 gm., Benincasa hispida seeds 25 gm., Coix lachryma-jobi kernels 15 gm., Prunus persica kernels 6 gm., as decoction.

2. Febrile illness, dryness in mouth and tongue: Use the "Five-juice drink": Take Phragmites rhizomes, pear, water chest-nut, lotus roots, and sugar cane (or Liriope spicata tubers), all in the fresh state, mash to obtain juice. Mix the juices and take warm or cold.

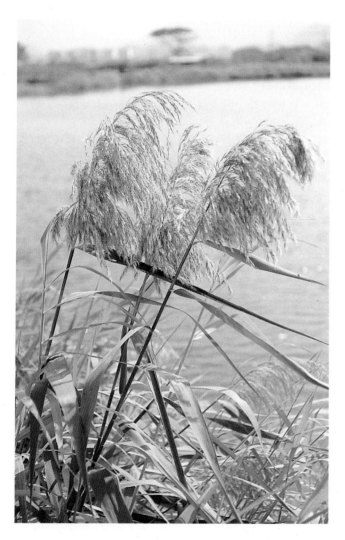

　　禾本科、蘆葦屬之多年生草本，根狀莖粗壯。稈高1至3米。圓錐花序頂生，長10至40厘米，分枝斜向上生長或微向外伸展；小穗常包含4至7朵小花，第一朵小花常為雄性。由根狀莖向四周延生，長成極大片之蘆葦羣落，於大量開花時，極易判別出本種。花期：九月至十月。

Gramineae: Perennial herbs, rhizomes stout, culms 1-3m high. Panicles terminal, 10-40cm long, inflorescence branches oblique or slightly extending outwards; spikelets usually consisting of 4-7 florets, the first one usually male. Rhizomes spreading in all directions to form a vast colony. The plant is easily distinguished when in profuse bloom. Flowering from September to October.

南 蛇 棒

Amorphophallus dunnii Tutcher

別　　名　鄧氏蒟蒻。

生長環境　生於土壤肥沃的林下陰濕處。

採集加工　藥用塊莖。夏、秋季採挖，除去地上莖葉及鬚根，放陰涼處風乾。

性味功能　味辛，性寒。有毒。消腫散結，解毒止痛。

主治用法　腫瘤，頸淋巴結結核，癰癤腫毒，蛇咬傷。每用3至5錢，水煎服。大量可以用至1兩（但須煎3小時後才能服用）；外用適量，搗爛敷患處。

Habitat　　　In thick, fertile soil under woods, and on damp, shady sites.

Preparation　　Use tubers. Collect in summer and autumn, discard the rootlets and the leaves and stem which appear above ground level, dry under shade.

Properties　　Acrid tasting; cold, toxic. Resolves swelling; anti-inflammatory, analgesic.

Indications　　Tumour, tuberculous adenitis, furuncles and carbuncles, snake bites. Use 10-15 gm., as decoction. For external use, mash fresh herb and apply to the lesion.

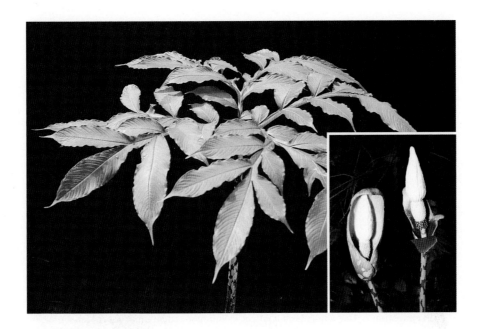

　　天南星科、魔芋屬之多年生草本，塊莖扁球形，密生分枝肉質根。鱗葉多數，綫形，膜質。葉片3全裂，裂片離基10厘米以上2次分叉，小裂片互生；葉柄長，乾時綠白色，具暗綠色小斑。花序柄顏色與葉柄同；佛焰苞綠色或淺綠白色，乾時膜質，下部蓆捲，內部黃綠色而基部紫色；肉穗花序短於佛焰苞；附屬器長圓錐形，頂端鈍圓，具綠色及黃白色。漿果藍色。花期：三月至四月。

　　Araceae: Perennial herbs, tuber compressed globose, succulent branching roots numerous. Scale leaves numerous, linear, membranous. Leaf trifoliolate, each leaflet divided twice into two lobes 10cm from the base, lobes alternate; long-petiolate; petiole and rachis greenish-white when dry, with dark green patches. Scape same colour as the leaves. Spathe green or light greenish-white, membranous when dry, rolling below, inner surface yellowish-green, purple at base; spadix shorter than spathe; appendage linear conic, apex obtuse, green or yellowish-white. Berry blue. Flowering from March to April.

芋

Colocasia esculenta (L.) Schott

別　　名　芋頭、芋艿、芋魁、土芝、蹲鴟。

生長環境　多為栽培，或逸生於濕地。

採集加工　藥用全株。夏、秋採收，曬乾或鮮用。

性味功能　味甘、辛，性平。塊莖（芋頭）：有小毒，消炎，散結。葉、葉柄：解毒，收斂。

主治用法　芋頭：瘰癧，癰瘡腫毒。每用2至4兩，水煎服。葉柄：蕁麻疹，腹瀉。每用5錢至2兩。葉治蜂螫傷。全株外用治瘡癬，鮮品搗敷患處。

方　　例　1. 瘰癧（淋巴結結核）：陳海蜇、荸薺各500克，煎濃汁，和芋頭粉500克，製成藥丸，每次服3至5克，每日服三次。

2. 蕁麻疹：芋葉柄1至2兩，同豬排骨燉服。

主要成分　芋頭含澱粉69.6-73.7%，蛋白質1.75-2.3%，脂類0.47-0.68%，以及維他命 B_1、B_2 等，並含氰甙。

附　　註　芋頭生用有小毒，煮熟可作糧食，多食會滯脹。

Habitat　　Mostly cultivated (as taro). Sometimes found growing wild on damp soil.

Preparation　　Use whole herb. Collect in summer and autumn, dry under sun or use fresh.

Properties　　Sweet and acrid tasting; neutral. Rhizome (taro): Slightly toxic, anti-inflammatory; reduces swelling. Leaves and stalk: Anti-inflammatory, astringent.

Indications　　Rhizome: Scrofula, furuncles and carbuncles. Use 60-120 gm., as decoction. Leaf stalk: Urticaria, diarrhea. Use 15-60 gm. Leaves: bee-sting. The mashed fresh whole herb is used as poultice for boils.

Prescriptions　　1. Scrofula: Water chestnut, dried Rhopilema esculenta (edible jelly fish), 500 gm. each, heat together to obtain a thick sauce, add 500 gm. of taro powder to the sauce, and make into pills. Take three times daily, each time using 3-5 gm.

2. Urticaria: Leaf stalk of Colocasia esculenta, 30-60 gm., cook with pork spare ribs for consumption.

Remarks　　While taro is edible after cooking, it is slightly poisonous in the raw state. Too much intake results in indigestion and distention.

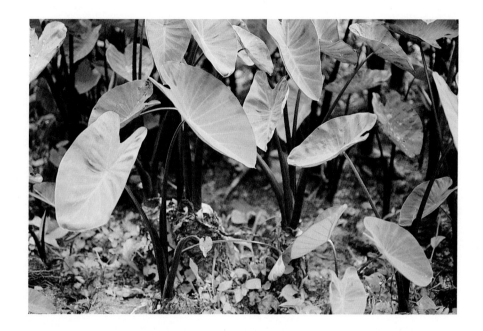

　　天南星科、芋屬之多年生草本。地下莖為卵形至長橢圓形，有豐富澱粉之褐色塊莖，具纖毛。葉基生，常4至5片簇生；葉片闊大，卵狀廣橢圓心形；質厚；葉緣帶波狀；葉面具防火性；葉柄粗長，肉質，綠色或淡綠紫色，基部呈鞘狀。花莖1至4枝，自葉鞘基部抽出；佛焰苞淡黃色；肉穗花序長橢圓形，短於佛焰苞，上半部生多數黃色雄花，中部生中性花，下半部生綠色雌花。花期：二月至四月。

　　Araceae: Perennial herbs. Stem-tuber ovate to long elliptic, rich in starch, villose. Leaves basal, 4-5, clustered, large, broad ovate-cordate; thick; margin undulate; upper surface water-proof; petiole long and thick, succulent, green or pale greenish-purple, base sheath-like. Scapes 1-4, arising from base of leaf-sheath; spathe light yellow; spadix long elliptic, shorter than spathe, upper part with yellowish staminates, middle part with neutral flowers, lower part with greenish pistillates. Flowering from February to April.

藍 耳 草

Cyanotis vaga (Lour.) Roem. et Schult.

別　　名　如意草、雞冠參、露水草。

生長環境　生於山野、路旁。

採集加工　藥用根或全草。夏、秋採集，曬乾或鮮用。

性味功能　味甘、苦，性平。補虛，除濕，舒筋活絡。

主治用法　1. 體虛，虛熱不退；2. 腎炎水腫；3. 風濕性關節疼痛；4. 濕疹。每用 3 至 5 錢，水煎服。外用適量，鮮品搗爛敷患處。

方　　例　1. 虛熱不退：藍耳草根、盤龍參各5錢，水煎服，或本品煮瘦肉吃。

2. 風濕性關節痛：藍耳草根 5 錢泡酒服，或本品煮鱔魚吃。

主要成分　葉含 β - 蛻皮甾酮和環四十烷。

附　　註　外國有用本品來治療乳腺癌。

Habitat　　　In the open, or along roadside.

Preparation　　Use roots or whole herb. Collect in summer and autumn, dry under sun or use fresh.

Properties　　Sweet and bitter tasting; neutral. Tonic, anti-rheumatic; relaxes muscles, promotes circulation.

Indications　　1. Body weakness, prolonged low fever; 2. Nephritic edema; 3. Rheumatic arthralgia; 4. Eczema. Use 9-15 gm., as decoction. External use by mashing fresh herb as poultice.

Prescriptions　　1. Prolonged low fever; Cyanotis vaga roots, Spiranthes sinensis, 15 gm. each, as decoction. Or cook Cyanotis vaga with lean pork for food.

2. Rheumatic arthralgia: Cyanotis vaga roots 15 gm., steep in wine for consumption.

Remarks　　This herb has been used in some countries for the treatment of breast cancer.

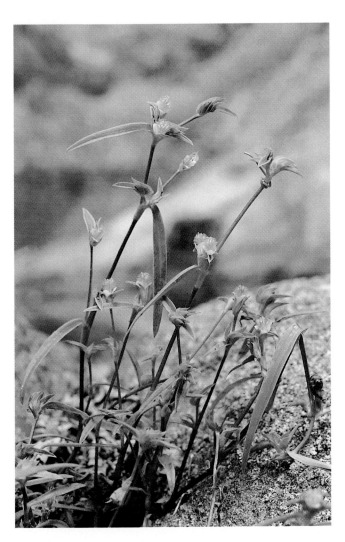

鴨跖草科、藍耳草屬之多年生披散草本，植株多少被疏長綿毛，高15至30厘米，鱗莖球狀，被毛。葉片披針形，長5至10厘米，寬0.5至2厘米，互生，葉緣具睫毛。總苞片比葉略寬、短，苞片鐮刀狀，兩列，每列覆瓦狀排列；萼片基部連合，披針形，外被白色綿毛；花瓣3片，藍色或紫藍色，中部合生成筒；雄蕊6，花絲上部被毛。蒴果倒卵狀三棱形，頂端被細長硬毛。花期：九月至十月。

Commelinaceae: Perennial diffuse herbs, more or less villose, 15-30cm high. Bulbs globular, hairy. Leaves alternate, lanceolate, 5-10cm long, 0.5-2cm wide, margin ciliate. Involucral bracts slightly wider and shorter than the leaves, falcate, imbricate, 2-ranked; calyx united at base, lanceolate, villose outside; petals 3, blue or purplish-blue, united in the middle to form a tube; stamens 6, upper portion of filament hairy. Capsules obovoid-trigonous, apex strigose. Flowering from September to October.

水葫蘆（水浮蓮）

Eichhornia crassipes (Mart.) Solms

別　　名　　大水萍、鳳眼蓮、鳳眼藍、洋水仙。

生長環境　　生於池塘和河溝中。

採集加工　　藥用全草。夏、秋採收，洗淨，曬乾或鮮用。

性味功能　　味淡，性涼。清熱利尿。

主治用法　　1. 中暑煩渴；2. 腎炎水腫，小便不利。每用 5 錢至 1 兩，水煎服。外用治瘡癤，鮮品適量，搗爛敷患處。

主要成分　　全草含二氧化硅、鈣、鎂、鉀、鈉、銅、錳、鐵等。葉含胡蘿蔔素。花含飛燕草素 -3- 二葡萄糖甙。

附　　註　　珠江一帶農民把本品作家畜飼料。馬來西亞有些人取其嫩葉、葉柄和花煮熟作蔬菜食用。本品對金黃色葡萄球菌、白喉桿菌、傷寒桿菌等均有抑制作用。

Habitat　　In ponds and streams.

Preparation　　Use whole herb. Collect in summer and autumn, wash, dry under sun or use fresh.

Properties　　Bland tasting; cool. Anti-inflammatory, diuretic.

Indications　　1. Heatstroke; 2. Nephritic edema, difficulty of urination. Use 15-30 gm., as decoction. External use for furuncles, by mashing fresh herb for topical application.

Remarks　　This herb is used by peasants in the Pearl River area as feeds for domestic animals. Inhabitants in some parts of Malaysia cook the young leaves, stalks, and flowers as vegetable. It is bacteriostatic against Staph. aureus, Diphtheria bacilli, and S. typhosa.

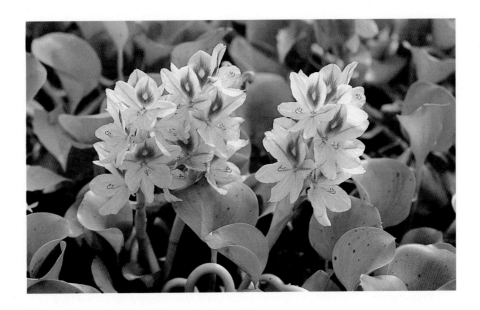

　　雨久花科、鳳眼蓮屬之浮水草本或根生於泥中，高 30 至 50 厘米。莖極短，具長匍匐枝，易與母株分離而另生新植株。葉基生，蓮座狀，寬卵形或菱形，長寬均約 2.5 至 12 厘米，葉尖圓鈍，葉基淺心形、截形、圓形或寬楔形，全緣，光亮，具弧狀脈；葉柄長短不一，長可達 30 厘米，中部膨脹成囊狀，內有氣室，基部有鞘狀包片。花葶多棱角；花多數，穗狀花序；花被裂片6，丁香紫色，上裂片之周圍藍色，中央有一黃斑。蒴果卵形。花期：夏季至秋季。

Pontederiaceae: Aquatic perennial herbs, 30-50cm high; floating or with creeping stems in mud. Stem very short, possessing long stolons which can easily separate from plant proper to establish new plants. Leaves basal, forming a rosette, broad ovate or rhombic, 2.5-12cm long and wide, apex obtuse, base shallowly cordate, truncate, round or broad cuneate, margin entire, shiny, veins arcuate; petioles variable, up to 30cm long, enlarged and spongy at middle, sheathy at basal end. Scapes ribbed; flowers numerous, forming a spike inflorescence; perianth segments 6, lilac-coloured, the upper segment having a yellow central patch surrounded by a blue rim. Capsules ovoid. Flowering from summer to autumn.

忽　地　笑

Lycoris aurea (L'Her.) Herb.

別　　名　黃花石蒜、大一枝箭、脫衣換錦、巖大蒜、鐵色箭。

生長環境　多栽培於庭園。

採集加工　藥用鱗莖。春、秋採挖，去苗葉，鮮用或切片曬乾。

性味功能　味辛，性平。有小毒。解毒，袪痰，催吐。

主治用法　1. 癰瘡腫毒；2. 耳下紅腫；3. 燙火傷。多作外用，鮮品適量搗敷，或絞汁外塗患處。本品有毒，內服宜慎。

方　　例　1. 癰瘡腫毒，耳下紅腫：忽地笑、野菊葉、馬藍，搗敷患處。

2. 燙火傷：忽地笑搗汁，和雞蛋清塗患處。

主要成分　鱗莖含石蒜鹼（lycorine）0.2%、加蘭他敏（galanthamin）、偽石蒜鹼等。

附　　註　全株有毒，以鱗莖最毒。中毒症狀為：流涎、嘔吐、瀉下、舌硬直、驚厥、手腳發冷、脈弱、休克。早期可飲濃茶、淡鹽水、洗胃等方法解救。

Habitat　　　Mostly cultivated in gardens.

Preparation　　Use bulbs. Collect in spring and autumn, discard leaves, use fresh or slice and dry under sun.

Properties　　Acrid tasting; neutral. Slightly toxic. Anti-inflammatory, expectorant, emetic.

Indications　　1. Carbuncles and furuncles; 2. subauricular swelling; 3. Scalds. Mostly used externally, mash fresh herb for local application, or squeeze to obtain juice for application. This herb is toxic; precaution should be observed when taking orally.

Prescriptions　　1. Furuncles and carbuncles, subauricular swelling: Lycoris aurea, Chrysanthemum indicum leaves, Strobilanthes cusia, mash and apply to lesion.

2. Scalds: Lycoris aurea, mash to obtain juice, then mix with egg white and apply to lesion.

Remarks　　The whole herb is poisonous. Signs of intoxication are: salivation, vomiting, diarrhea, stiff tongue, convulsion, cold extremities, weak pulse, shock. Antidote at an early stage consists of using concentrated tea, dilute salt solution, and gastric lavage.

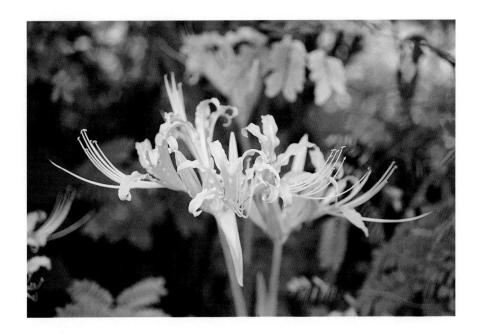

　　石蒜科、石蒜屬之多年生草本。鱗莖肥大，近球形，直徑約5厘米，外有黑褐色鱗莖皮。葉基生，質厚，寬長條形，上部漸次變狹，葉頂端圓形，葉片長達60厘米；葉面黃綠色，有光澤，葉背灰綠色；中脈在葉面凹下，在葉背隆起；葉脈及葉片基部帶紫紅色。先花後葉，花葶自鱗莖中央抽出，傘形花序有花5至10朵；花黃或橙色；花被筒裂片6，邊緣稍皺曲；雌雄蕊伸出花外。蒴果。花期：十月。

Amaryllidaceae: Perennial herbs. Bulb large, subglobose, 5cm across, external scale-leaves black-brown. Leaves basal, thick, broad-linear, up to 60cm long, gradually attenuate, apex obtuse; yellowish green above, glossy, pale-green beneath; midrib sunken on the upper and elevated on the lower surface; veins and leaf base scarlet. Flowers appearing before the leaves, yellow or orange, 5-10 in an umbel at the end of a scape which arises from the centre of the bulb; perianth segments 6, margin slightly wrinkled; stamens and pistils exserted. Fruits capsular. Flowering in October.

薑　黃

Curcuma longa L.

別　　名　黃薑、黃絲鬱金、寶鼎香。

生長環境　多為栽培。

採集加工　藥用根狀莖。冬季或初春採挖，煮熟，撞去外皮，或鮮品切片，曬乾。

性味功能　味辛、苦，性溫。行氣，破瘀，通經，止痛。

主治用法　1. 胸脅刺痛，肩臂痹痛；2. 月經不調，痛經，閉經；3. 跌打損傷。每用1至3錢，水煎服。外用適量。孕婦慎服。

方　　例　1. 肩臂痹痛：薑黃3錢，當歸、赤芍、海桐皮、白朮各2錢，生薑、薑活、炙甘草各1錢，水煎服。

2. 月經不調，痛經：薑黃、白芍、延胡索、丹皮、當歸各3錢，紅花、川芎各2錢，水煎服。

主要成分　根狀莖含薑黃素（curcumin）約0.3%、揮發油約1-5%，油中主要成分為薑黃酮（tumerone）、二氫薑黃酮50%、薑烯（zingiberen）20%等。

附　　註　薑黃為香港新記錄植物。

Habitat　　Mostly cultivated.

Preparation　　Use rhizome. Collect in winter or early spring, cook and remove the skin, or slice fresh rhizome, dry under sun.

Properties　　Acrid and bitter tasting; warm. Promotes circulation of "qi", reduces bruises, regulates menses; analgesic.

Indications　　1. Chest and rib pain, pain and numbness of arm and shoulder; 2. Irregular menses, dysmenorrhea, amenorrhea; 3. Traumatic injury. Use 3-10 gm., as decoction. Use sufficient amount topically. Contraindicated in pregnancy.

Prescription　　Arm and shoulder pain and numbness: Curcuma longa 10 gm., Angelica sinensis, Paeonia veitchii, Erythrina indica bark, Atractylodes macrocephala, 6 gm. each, Zingiber officinale, Notopterygium incisum, Glycyrrhiza uralensis, 3 gm. each, as decoction.

Remarks　　Curcuma longa is a newly recorded species in Hong Kong.

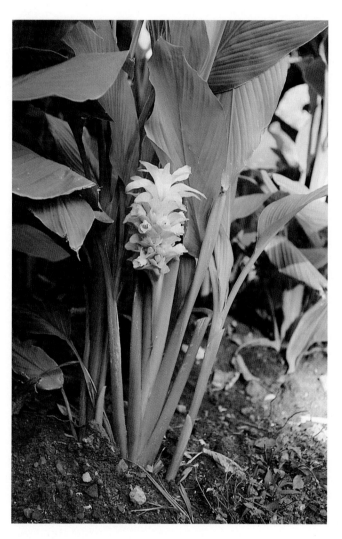

薑科、薑黃屬之多年生草本。根狀莖深黃色，極芳香。根粗壯，末端膨大。葉片大塊，矩圓形至橢圓形，葉柄約與葉片等長。穗狀花序圓柱狀，長12至15厘米，生於由葉鞘內抽出之花葶頂端；苞片卵形，綠白色，在每一苞片內有花多朵，上部無花的苞片較狹，頂端紅色；花冠管比花萼長2倍多；側生退化雄蕊與花絲基部相連；唇瓣倒卵形，白色，中部黃色；子房被微柔毛。花期：秋季。

Zingiberaceae: Perennial herbs. Rhizomes deep yellow, aromatic. Roots stout, swollen at the ends. Leaves large, oblong to elliptic, petioles and blades similar in length. Spike cylindrical, 12-15cm long, borne terminally at the end of a scape which arises from within the leaf sheaths; bracts ovate, greenish white, several flowers inside each bract, upper bracts without flowers, narrower, apex red; corolla tube more than 2 times longer than calyx; lateral staminodes and filament connate; lip obovate, white, yellow at middle; ovary pilose. Flowering in autumn.

山奈（沙薑）

Kaempferia galanga L.

別　　名　三奈、三賴、三奈子、山辣。

生長環境　多為栽培。

採集加工　藥用根狀莖。冬季採收，剪去鬚根，切片曬乾。

性味功能　味辛，性溫。溫中健胃，消食止痛。

主治用法　1. 胃寒疼痛，飲食不消；2. 急性胃腸炎，腹痛泄瀉；3. 牙痛，跌打損傷。每用2至3錢，水煎服。外用粉末適量，塞齲齒中或擦牙。本品亦常用作調味品。

方　　例　1. 胃寒冷痛：沙薑、丁香、當歸、甘草等分為末，醋糊丸如梧桐子大。每服 30 丸，酒送服。

2. 感冒食滯，腹痛泄瀉：沙薑 5 錢，豆豉薑根 2 錢，南五味子根 3 錢，烏藥 1 錢 5 分，陳茶葉 1 錢。研末，每次 5 錢，開水泡或煎數沸後取汁服。

主要成分　含揮發油、黃酮、香豆素、蛋白質、澱粉、黏液質等。

Habitat　　　Mostly cultivated.

Preparation　　Use rhizomes. Collect in winter, remove the rootlets, slice and dry under sun.

Properties　　Acrid tasting; warm. Stomachic; promotes digestion; analgesic.

Indications　　1. Gastric pain, indigestion; 2. Acute gastroenteritis, stomachache, diarrhea; 3. Toothache, traumatic injury. Use 5-10 gm., as decoction. External use of pulverized herb in dental caries, or for brushing the teeth. This herb is also commonly used as a spice.

Prescriptions　　1. Stomachache: Kaempferia galanga, Eugenia caryophyllata, Angelica sinensis, Glycyrrhiza uralensis, in equal amounts as powder. Mix with vinegar to make pellets with a size of that of Firmiana simplex seeds (about 5mm diameter). Take 30 pellets each time with wine.

2. Common colds, indigestion, stomachache and diarrhea: Kaempferia galanga 15 gm., Litsea cubeba root 6 gm., Kadsura coccinea root 10 gm., Lindera aggregata 5 gm., Camellia sinensis 3 gm., grind into powder, take 15 gm. each time with water.

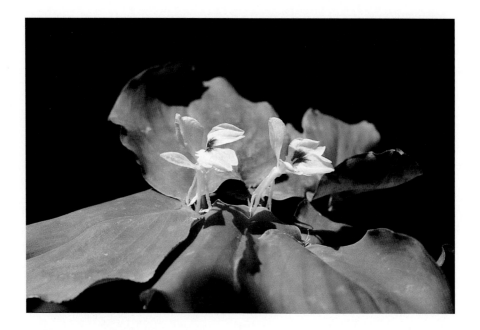

　　薑科、山柰屬之多年生草本。根狀莖塊狀，芳香。葉片近圓形，平行脈，葉頂端闊漸尖；2至4片貼近地面生長；無毛或於葉背被稀疏之長柔毛，乾燥時之葉面可見紅色小點；近無葉柄；葉鞘長2至3厘米。花白色，有香味，易凋；6至12朵頂生，半藏於葉鞘中；花冠管之裂片條形；側生退化雄蕊倒卵狀楔形；唇瓣深2裂至中部以下，基部具紫斑；雄蕊無花絲。花期：七月至九月。

Zingiberaceae: Perennial herbs. Rhizomes tuberous, aromatic. Leaves suborbicular, parallel veined, apex broadly acuminate; 2-4 near the ground; glabrous or sparsely villose beneath, small red dots above when dry; subsessile, leaf sheath 2-3cm long. Flowers white, fragrant, 6-12 terminal, withering early; half of the flower concealed inside the leaf sheath; corolla tube segments linear; lateral staminodes obovate-cuneiform; lip deeply two-lobed, base with purple patches; filaments none. Flowering from July to September.

珊 瑚 薑

Zingiber corallinum Hance

生長環境　生於近海密林中。

採集加工　藥用根狀莖。夏、秋採收，切片曬乾。

性味功能　味辛，性溫。消腫解毒。

主治用法　1. 風濕骨痛；2. 跌打骨折。每用 3 至 5 錢，水煎服。外用鮮品搗爛敷患處，外加夾板包紮固定。

附　　註　珊瑚薑為香港的新記錄植物。

Habitat　　　In woods near the sea.

Preparation　Use rhizome. Collect in summer and autumn, wash, slice, sun-dry.

Properties　Acrid tasting; neutral. Anti-swelling, anti-inflammatory.

Indications　1. Rheumatic joint pain; 2. Traumatic fracture. Dose is 10-15 gm., as decoction. External use with mashed fresh herb as poultice, plus splinting.

Remarks　　This is a newly recorded species in Hong Kong.

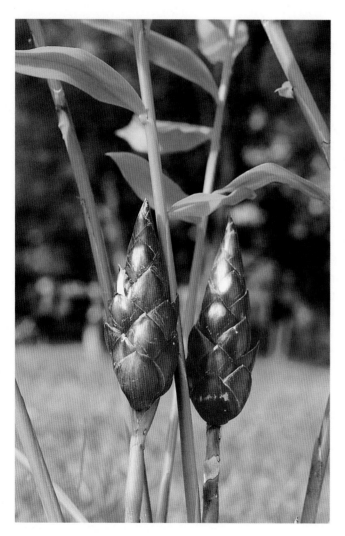

薑科、薑屬之多年生有香味草本，高約1米。葉2行排列，葉片長圓狀披針形至披針形，葉鞘張開。穗狀花序長圓形，總花梗被鱗片狀鞘；苞片卵形，紅色，頂端急尖；花萼管膜質，沿一側開裂幾達中部；花冠裂片紅色，長圓形，漸尖，後方的一枚較寬；唇瓣中央裂片倒卵形；花絲缺如，花藥之基部藏於花冠管內；子房被絹毛。種子黑色而光亮，假種皮白色、撕裂狀。花期：五月至八月。

Zingiberaceae: Perennial aromatic herbs, about 1m high. Leaves distichous, blade oblong-lanceolate to lanceolate, leaf sheath open. Spike inflorescence cylindrical, peduncle covered by scale-like sheaths; bract ovate, red, apex acute; calyx tube membranous, splitting along one side almost to the middle; corolla lobes red, petals oblong-orbicular, acuminate, the posterior one wider; the middle lobe of the labellum obovate; filaments none, the bases of anthers enclosed within corolla tube; ovary covered with silky hairs. Seeds black, glossy, aril white, lacerating. Flowering from May to August.

蘘　荷

Zingiber mioga (Thunb.) Rosc.

別　　名　　苴蓴、土裏開花、野山薑、蓮花薑。

生長環境　　生於山坡林邊、溪溝旁等陰濕處。

採集加工　　藥用根狀莖。夏、秋採收，洗淨，曬乾或鮮用。

性味功能　　味辛，性溫。溫中健胃，活血止痛。

主治用法　　1. 胃痛，腹痛；2. 腰腿痛；3. 跌打損傷。每用3錢至5錢，水煎服。有胃出血者忌服。外用治癰瘡腫毒，鮮品適量搗爛敷患處或煎水外洗。

方　　例　　1. 腰腿痛：蘘荷5錢，豬瘦肉4兩，水燉，服湯食肉。

2. 胃痛：蘘荷5錢，水煎服。或開裂的果實3至4兩，白糖適量，水煎服。

主要成分　　根莖含α-蒎烯（α-pinene）、β-蒎烯、β-水芹烯（β-phellandrene）。

附　　註　　蘘荷為香港的新記錄植物。

Habitat　　On slopes, edges of woods, creek banks and in damp shady areas.

Preparation　　Use rhizomes. Collect in summer and autumn, wash, dry, or use fresh.

Properties　　Acrid tasting; warm. Stomachic; promotes circulation; analgesic.

Indications　　1. Gastric pain, stomachache; 2. Loin pain; 3. Traumatic injury. Use 10-15 gm., as decoction. Contraindicated in cases with gastric haemorrhage. External use in boils and abscesses. Mash fresh herb and apply to lesion, or use for washing.

Prescriptions　　1. Loin and leg pain: Use Zingiber mioga 15 gm., cook with 120 gm. lean pork for consumption.

2. Epigastric pain: Use Zingiber mioga 15 gm., as decoction. May also use 90-120 gm. of fruits that have split open together with a suitable quantity of sugar as decoction.

Remarks　　Rhizome contains α-pinene, and β-phellandrene. This is a newly recorded species in Hong Kong.

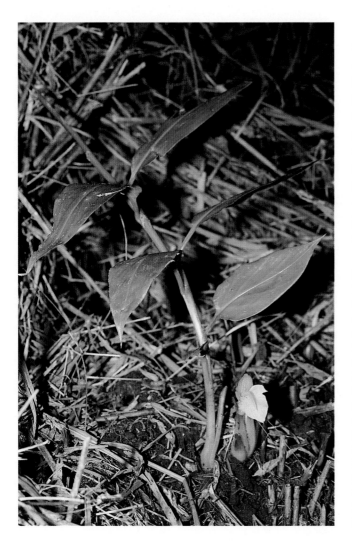

薑科、薑屬之多年生有香味草本，高約1米。根狀莖淡黃色，有辛辣味。植株基部有數枚無葉的鞘。葉片長圓狀披針形，兩面散生若干黑色小點；葉舌2裂、膜質。穗狀花序橢圓形，長5至7厘米，生於單獨發自根狀莖之花葶上；總花梗柔弱，被長圓形至披針形之鱗鞘；花萼管狀，佛焰苞狀開裂；花冠管略長於萼管，裂片披針形，白色；唇瓣淡黃色而中央較深色；子房被絹毛。蒴果卵形，3瓣裂。花期：八月至十月。

Zingiberaceae: Perennial aromatic herbs, about 1m high. Rhizomes light yellow, possessing an acrid taste. Base of the plant with several bladeless sheaths. Leaves oblong-lanceolate, a number of scattered black dots appearing on both surfaces; ligule 2 lobed, membranous. Spike ellipsoidal, 5-7cm long, solitary on a scape which arises from the rhizome; peduncle delicate, covered with scale-sheaths which are oblong-orbicular to lanceolate; calyx tubular, opening in the shape of a spathe; corolla tube slightly longer than calyx tube, lobes lanceolate, white; labellum (lip) light yellow, deeper at centre; ovary sericious. Fruits capsular, opening into 3 valves. Flowering from August to October.

薑（生薑）

Zingiber officinale Rosc.

別　　名　薑皮、乾薑、炮薑。

生長環境　多為栽培。

採集加工　藥用根狀莖。秋、冬採挖，除去莖葉和鬚根，多鮮用；其栓皮名生薑皮，乾燥品名乾薑，炒製後發泡鼓起，名炮薑。

性味功能　味辛，性微溫。發汗解表，健胃止嘔，化痰止咳，解毒。

主治用法　1. 風寒感冒；2. 胃寒嘔吐；3. 寒痰咳嗽。每用 1 至 3 錢，水煎服。生薑可解半夏、南星毒。

方　　例　1. 風寒感冒：生薑 5 片，紫蘇葉 1 兩，水煎服。

2. 胃寒嘔吐：生薑、半夏各 3 錢，水煎服。

主要成分　含揮發油、酚性物質、糖、多種氨基酸等。

附　　註　生薑皮：味辛，性微溫；利水消腫。乾薑：味辛，性熱；溫中健胃，回陽通脈。炮薑：味辛，性熱；溫經止血。

Habitat　　　Mostly cultivated (as ginger).

Preparation　　Use rhizome. Collect in autumn and winter, remove leaves and rootlets, use fresh.

Properties　　Acrid tasting; slightly warm. Diaphoretic, stomachic, antiemetic, expectorant and antitussive, anti-inflammatory.

Indications　　1. Rheumatism and common cold; 2. Stomachache and vomiting; 3. Productive coughs. Use 3-10 gm., as decoction. Zingiber could be used as antidote for poisoning by Arisaema (erubescens) and Pinellia (ternata).

Prescriptions　　1. Common cold: Zingiber officinale 5 slices, Perilla frutescens leaves 30 gm., as decoction.

2. Stomach discomfort and vomiting: Zingiber officinale, Pinellia ternata, 10 gm. each, as decoction.

Remarks　　Skin of fresh ginger: Acrid and warm; diuretic. Dried ginger: Acrid, hot; warms the stomach, promotes circulation. Roasted ginger: Acrid and hot; haemostatic.

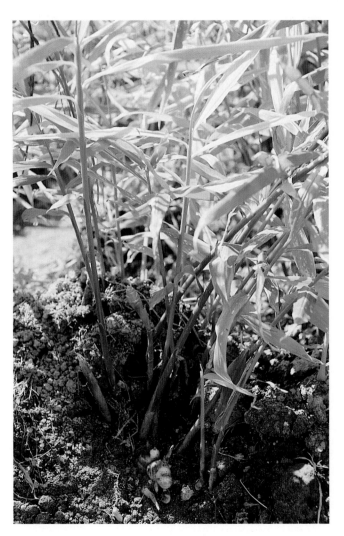

　　薑科、薑屬之多年生草本，高可達 1 米。根狀莖肉質、肥厚，有芳香及辛辣味。葉片長披針形，長 15 至 30 厘米，寬約 2.5 厘米；葉舌膜質。花葶單獨自根莖抽出；穗狀花序卵形；苞片淡綠色，頂端有小尖頭；花冠管黃綠色，裂片披針形，長不及 2 厘米；唇瓣中央裂片矩圓狀倒卵形，短於花冠裂片，有紫色條紋及淡黃色斑點，側裂片卵形；花藥之藥隔附屬體包裹着花柱。花期：秋季。

Zingiberaceae: Perennial herbs, up to 1m high. Rhizomes fleshy, large, aromatic and acrid. Leaves linear-lanceolate, 15-30cm long, about 2.5cm wide; ligule membranous. Scape solitary, emerging from the rhizome; spike ovoid; bract light green, tip mucronate; corolla tube yellowish green, lobes lanceolate, shorter than 2cm; central lobe of lip orbicular-obovate, shorter than corolla lobes, with purple stripes and light yellow spots, lateral lobes ovate; style enclosed by appendage of the connective of the anther. Flowering in autumn.

陽　荷

Zingiber striolatum Diels

別　　名　野薑。

生長環境　生於山谷林下陰濕處。

採集加工　藥用根狀莖。秋、冬季可採，切片曬乾。

性味功能　味辛，性溫。溫中健胃，止痛。

主治用法　胃痛，腹痛。每用 1 錢至 3 錢，水煎服。

附　　註　陽荷為香港的新記錄植物。

Habitat　　　In ravines, under woods, on moist areas.

Preparation　Use rhizome. Collect in autumn and winter, slice and dry under sun.

Properties　Acrid tasting; warm. Stomachic, analgesic.

Indications　Epigastric pain, abdominal pain. Use 3-10 gm., as decoction.

Remarks　This is a newly recorded species in Hong Kong.

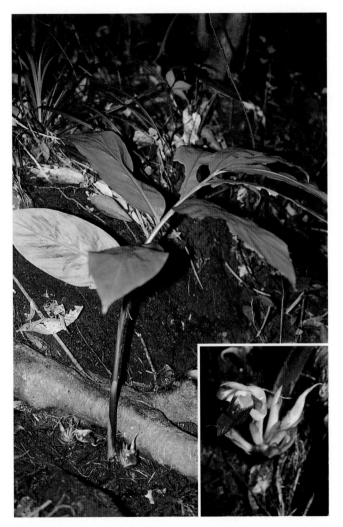

薑科、薑屬之多年生草本，高約 1 米。根狀莖白色，略有芳香味。葉片橢圓狀披針形至披針形，葉背分佈極疏之柔毛至無毛；葉舌膜質，2 裂，具褐色條紋。總花梗被 2 至 3 枚鱗片；花序近卵形，苞片紅色，寬卵形或橢圓形，被疏柔毛；花萼膜質；花冠管白色，長 4 至 6 厘米，裂片白或稍帶黃色，有紫褐色條紋；唇瓣倒卵形，淺紫色；花絲極短。蒴果熟時 3 瓣開裂，內果皮紅色。花期：七月至九月。

Zingiberaceae: Perennial herbs, about 1m high. Rhizomes white, slightly aromatic. Leaves elliptic-lanceolate to lanceolate, subglabrous to glabrous beneath; ligule membranous, 2-lobed, with brown stripes, 2-3 scales on peduncle; inflorescence subovoid, bracts red, broadly ovate or elliptic, sparsely pilose; calyx membranous; corolla tube white, 4-6cm long, lobes white or slightly tinged with yellow, with purple-brown stripes; lip obovate, light purple; filament very short. Fruits capsular, splitting into 3 valves on maturity, endocarp red. Flowering from July to September.

蕉　蘭

Acampe multiflora (Lindl.) Lindl.

別　　　名　多花脆蘭、黑山蔗。

生長環境　生於疏林的樹上或巖石上。

採集加工　藥用根、葉。全年可採，多鮮用。

性味功能　味辛、微苦，性平。活絡，止痛。

主治用法　治跌打損傷，骨折。每用2至5錢，水煎服。外用適量，鮮品搗爛敷患處。

Habitat　　　On trees and rocks in sparse forests.

Preparation　Use roots and leaves. Collect all year round, use fresh.

Properties　Acrid and bitter tasting; neutral. Promotes circulation; analgesic.

Indications　Traumatic injury, fractures. Use 6-15 gm., as decoction. For external use, mash fresh herb as poultice.

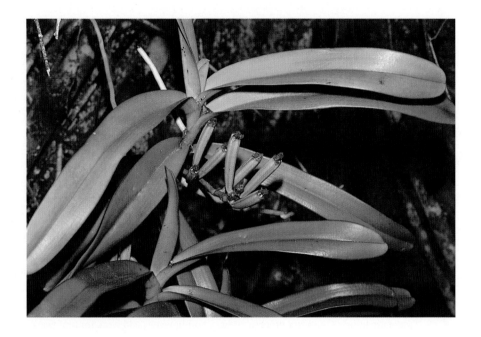

　　蘭科、脆蘭屬之多年生附生蘭。莖粗壯。葉肉質，多呈直立向上，帶狀矩圓形，長可達40厘米，闊約4厘米，葉尖為不等之2圓裂；平行葉脈。花莖直立，粗壯，約與葉等長，常具少數短分枝；花苞片質厚，三角形；花肉質，淡黃色帶紅色斑點及條紋；中萼片與側萼片約等大；花瓣較狹窄；唇瓣向上，矩圓形。蒴果明顯，長紡錘形或長矩圓形，長度可達8厘米。花期：九月至十月。

Orchidaceae: Perennial epiphytic orchid. Stems stout. Leaves fleshy, mostly erect, linear-oblong, up to 40cm long, 4cm wide; parellel venation; apex 2 unequal rounded lobes. Scapes erect, stout, about the same length as the leaves; often with branched short peduncles; bracts thick, deltoid; flowers fleshy, light yellow with red spots and stripes; dorsal sepal equals lateral sepals in size; petals narrower; lip erect, round. Capsule prominent, fusiform or oblong, up to 8cm in length. Flowering from September to October.

高 斑 葉 蘭

Goodyera procera (Ker-Gawl.) Hook.

別　　名　石風丹、山石竹、小芭蕉、蘭草花。

生長環境　生於溪澗濕地或附生於石壁上。

採集加工　藥用全草。冬季採挖，曬乾或鮮用。

性味功能　味辛、苦，性溫。祛風除濕，養血舒筋。

主治用法　1. 風濕關節痛，半身不遂；2. 跌打損傷；3. 支氣管炎，哮喘。每用 3 至 5 錢，水煎或浸酒服。孕婦忌服。

方　　例　1. 關節痛：高斑葉蘭 8 錢，豬腳 1 隻，水燉服。

2. 跌打損傷：高斑葉蘭 3 錢，水煎，加酒適量服。

Habitat　　　Thrives along creeks, streams, moist land, or on rock walls.

Preparation　Use whole herb. Collect in winter, dry under sun or use fresh.

Properties　Acrid and bitter tasting; warm. Anti-rheumatic, nourishing to the blood; relaxes the muscles.

Indications　1. Rheumatism, arthralgia, hemiplegia; 2. Traumatic injury; 3. Bronchitis, asthma. Use 10-15 gm., as decoction, or steep in wine. Contraindicated in pregnancy.

Prescriptions　1. Arthralgia: Goodyera procera 25 gm., cook with pork hock for consumption.

2. Traumatic injury: Goodyera procera 10 gm., boil in water, add wine for oral use.

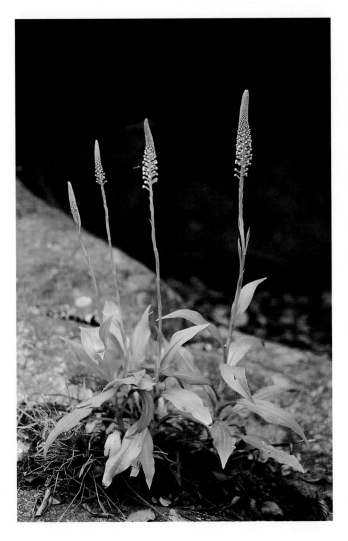

蘭科、斑葉蘭屬之多年生陸生蘭，高25至80厘米。根狀莖短；莖直立，有多片葉。葉長8至15厘米，寬2至5.5厘米，矩圓形或狹橢圓形，葉尖呈漸尖，葉基漸狹而成長而厚的柄。總狀花序頂生，其稠密的花，似穗狀，長10至15厘米；花苞片膜質，約與子房等長；花細小，白色而帶淡綠，芳香；萼片卵形；花瓣較狹，匙形，頂端略靠合；唇瓣囊狀，內面有柔毛，頂端鈍，向外反折，內有2枚胼胝體；合蕊柱短而闊；蕊喙2裂；花藥卵狀三角形。花期：四月至五月。

Orchidaceae: Perennial terrestrial orchids 25-80cm high. Rhizomes short. Leaves oblong-elliptic, 8-15cm long, 2-5.5cm wide, apex acuminate, base attenuate, petiolate. Flowers small, numerous, in dense terminal spike-like racemes 10-15cm long; bracts membranous, equal ovary in length; perianth white, tinged green, fragrant; sepals ovate, petals narrower, spatulate, apex slightly connivent; lip saccate, pilose inside, obtuse at the tip, reflexed, with 2 calli inside; column short, rostrum bifid; anthers ovate-deltoid. Flowering in April and May.

橙黃玉鳳花

Habenaria rhodocheila Hance

別　　名　紅人蘭、雞腎草、飛花羊。

生長環境　生於林下陰濕處或石上。

採集加工　藥用塊根。春、夏採收，曬乾或鮮用。

性味功能　味苦，性平。補腎，收斂。

主治用法　1. 腎虛腰痛；2. 陽萎，疝氣；3. 小兒遺尿。每用2至5錢，水煎服。外用治瘡瘍腫毒，跌打損傷，鮮品搗爛敷患處。

Habitat　　　　On damp soil under woods and on rocks.

Preparation　　Use tubers. Collect in spring and summer, dry under sun or use fresh.

Properties　　　Bitter tasting; neutral. Tonic to the "kidneys"; astringent.

Indications　　 1. Low back pain from weak "kidneys"; 2. Impotence, hernia; 3. Enuresis in children. Use 6-15 gm., as decoction. External use in pyodermas, traumatic injury, by applying mashed fresh herb as poultice.

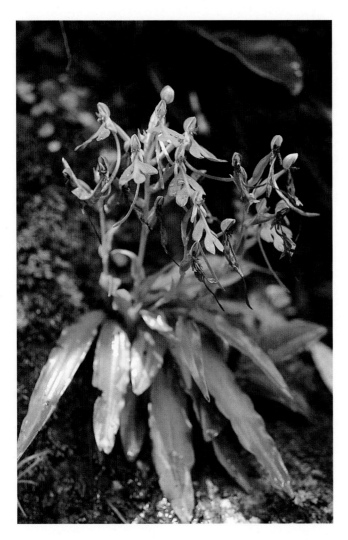

蘭科、玉鳳花屬之多年生、直立陸生蘭，高可達35厘米。塊莖長圓形，肉質。葉數片，長條狀矩圓形，漸尖，基部抱莖。總狀花序，疏生2至10數朵花；花苞片披針形；萼片綠色，中萼片半球形，側萼片矩圓形；花瓣綠色，直立，條狀匙形；唇瓣橙黃色，比萼片長2至3倍；距彎曲，黃色，較唇瓣幾長1倍；柱頭2裂，凸起物粗壯；子房纖細。花期：八月。

Orchidaceae: Perennial terrestrial erect orchids, up to 35cm high. Tuber cylindrical, fleshy. Leaves several, linear-oblong, apex acuminate, base amplexicaul. Flowers 2 to 10-plus in racemes; bracts lanceolate; sepals green, dorsal one semi-globose, lateral ones oblong; petals green, erect, linear-spatulate; labellum orange in colour, 2-3 times longer than the sepals; spur bent, yellow, almost twice as long as the labellum; stigma bifid, column stout; ovary delicate. Flowering in August.

鐮翅羊耳蒜

Liparis plicata Franch. et Sav.

別　　名　石海椒、石蓮草、果上葉。

生長環境　附生於山谷巖石上或林中樹上。

採集加工　藥用全草。春季採集，曬乾或鮮用。

性味功能　味甘，性平。清熱，止咳。

主治用法　1. 咳嗽；2. 小兒疳積、腹瀉。每用 5 錢至 1 兩，水煎服。

Habitat　　　Epiphytic on rocks or trees in ravines and woods.

Preparation　Use whole herb. Collect in spring, dry under sun or use fresh.

Properties　Sweet tasting; neutral. Anti-inflammatory, antitussive.

Indications　1. Coughs; 2. Infantile malabsorption, diarrhea. Use 15-30 gm., as decoction.

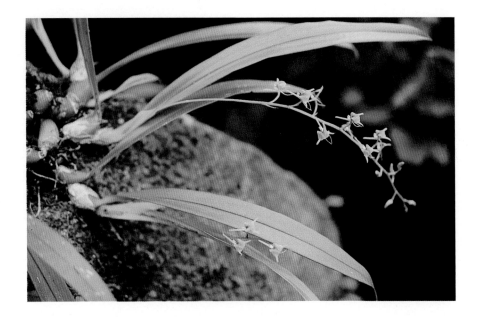

　　蘭科、羊耳蒜屬之附生蘭。假鱗莖狹矩圓形或卵狀圓錐形，只生一片葉。葉片近革質，狹矩圓形至倒披針形，長約11至20厘米，寬18至20毫米，葉尖呈急尖，葉基漸狹成柄，有關節。花葶約與葉等長，稍具翅；總狀花序長約為花莖的一半，花多數；花苞片狹披針形，短於花梗連子房；花淺褐色；中萼片狹披針形，稍反折，側萼片一對略平行；花瓣絲狀，下彎，等長於萼片；唇瓣楔狀矩圓形，具齒；合蕊柱彎曲，近端之蕊柱翅向下彎呈鐮刀狀。花期：十一月。

Orchidaceae: Epiphytic orchids. Pseudobulbs narrow-oblong or ovate-conic. Leaf 1, subcoriaceous, oblong-lanceolate, 11-20cm long, 18-20mm wide, apex acute, base attenuate, petiolate, articulate. Flowers greenish yellow, in terminal racemes on slightly winged scapes which are about as long as the leaves; bracts lanceolate, shorter than the ovary and pedicel together; flower light brown; dorsal sepal lanceolate, recurved, lateral sepals almost parallel; petals filiform, equal sepals in length, downward bending; lip cuneate-oblong, toothed; column curved, possessing falcate wings towards the apex. Flowering in November.

筆畫索引

207

INDEX

209

213

215

Index of English Common Names